THE Homeopathic EMERGENCY GUIDE

THE Homeopathic EMERGENCY GUIDE

A Quick Reference Handbook to Effective Homeopathic Care

THOMAS KRUZEL, N.D.

North Atlantic Books
Berkeley, California

Homeopathic Educational Services
Berkeley, California

The Homeopathic Emergency Guide

ISBN 1-55643-123-6

Published by
North Atlantic Books
P.O. Box 12327
Berkeley, California 94701–9998
and
Homeopathic Educational Services
2124 Kittredge Street
Berkeley, California 94704

Cover and book design by Paula Morrison

Printed in the United States of America by Malloy Lithographing

The Homeopathic Emergency Guide is sponsored by the Society for the Study of Native Arts and Sciences, a nonprofit educational corporation whose goals are to develop an educational and crosscultural perspective linking various scientific, social, and artistic fields; to nurture a holistic view of arts, sciences, humanities, and healing; and to publish and distribute literature on the relationship of mind, body, and nature.

Acknowledgements

This manuscript could not have been completed without the input and support of the following individuals. Their time and effort are sincerely appreciated. Steve Albin, N.D., John G. Collins, N.D., Durr Elmore, D.C., N.D., Paul Herscu, N.D., Tori Hudson, N.D., Ravinder Sahni, D. C., N.D. and Michael Traub, N.D., my first teachers of homeopathy both in the classroom and clinical setting. Krista Heron, N.D., Stephen King, N.D., Adam Ladd, N.D. and Steven Sandberg-Lewis, N.D., for manuscript review. Special thanks to Roger Morrison, M.D. for his suggestions for manuscript improvement and to Stephen Messer, N.D. for allowing the reproduction of his excellent flow charts.

Thanks also to Mitch Bebel, N.D., Mona Morstein, N.D. and Joan Ellen Macredis, N.D., for their assistance in manuscript preparation. Special thanks is extended to Paul Mittman, N.D. and Naturopathic Publications, without whose encouragement and patience this book would never have been published. My appreciation to Friedhelm Kirchfield and Medicina Biologica for providing their ongoing encouragement and support. Additionally I would like to thank Dana Ullman and North Atlantic Books for their continued advocacy of homeopathic medicine and assistance in making this current edition possible.

Lastly, I would like to thank Karen Banfield both for her help with manuscript review and for her ongoing, loving support.

Contents

Foreword

All cases of dynamic diseases, acute or chronic, even when resulting from mechanical or psychological injuries, are amenable to homeopathy, the science of therapeutics. By carefully applying the law of similars, the physician will observe that all cases of curable dynamic disease are curable with homeopathy. To achieve this noble goal the physician must be thoroughly familiar with the principles of homeopathy as taught in the ***Organon*** and must know how to make use of the reliable materia medica such as Hahnemann's ***Chronic Diseases***. Repertories are used as essential links between the patients symptoms and our vast materia medica.

Clinical guides such as this ***Homeopathic Emergency Guide***, provide the practitioner with a synopsis of the most characteristic symptoms of the leading remedies in a given condition. Their objective is to give assistance, especially to the less experienced practitioner, in those acute cases where long research for the simillimum is not always practical. Because these acute cases are often good opportunities for the younger practitioner to develop confidence in his/her skills and in homeopathy (as there is no context where the patient responds as quickly to the indicated remedy), this ***Homeopathic Emergency Guide*** will prove to be extremely helpful.

When using clinical guides it is important to be aware of two general drawbacks. First, any clinical guide fails through its inherent incompleteness because only leading remedies in a given condition can be presented. Also, the symptomology of each remedy presented is limited to only the leading characteristic symptoms. In clinical practice the patient will most of the time present some symptoms that can only be found in a more complete materia medica.

Second, there is the inevitable temptation to associate remedies ("the best remedies") with a given disease. The practice of pure homeopathy consists of constant individualization. The more we understand our science the more we individualize. Allopathy tends to treat the disease by generalizing. Such and such drugs are identified with a class of disease and vice versa. In homeopathy our aim is to restore health by treating the sick through constant individualization. Any remedy could be indicated in any given case even if never reported or suggested before. This unlimited possibility of making the best correspondence between the symptoms of the patient and the remedy, as required by the law of similars, is denied to us in the clinical guide. It is important to understand that for the practice of homeopathy it is not essential to know the name of the disease and, in fact, the more pathognomonic a symptom is, the less value it has for finding the indicated remedy. However it is different for allopathy where the diagnosis of a pathological entity is usually essential for the administration of the treatment. Nonetheless the knowledge of pathology and diagnosis remains as important for the homeopath as it is for the allopath but for different purposes. Adolph Lippe, the great homeopathic master, wrote that "the more knowledge the healer has of pathology the better will he be able to discern these very characteristic and valuable symptoms essentially belonging to the individual and not to the sick physiology, *therefore* the best pathologist will make the best healer."

Hahnemann developed homeopathy during a period of over 50 years. He never published any of his clinical cases or came close to writing a clinical guide. He was very adamant about not associating remedies with the name of a disease. In fact he was greatly annoyed when Franz Hartmann, one of his closest students, published in 1831 ***Therapeutics of Acute Diseases***. In this clinical guide Hartmann had attempted to facilitate the practice of homeopathy for beginners and for allopaths by associating remedies with names of diseases. Hahnemann wrote at once to Hartmann the following: "Owing to the difficult nature of our homeopathic method of treatment, which requires so much thought and subtle differentiation for it to be successfully practiced, to try and popularize and render it empirical to the extent you intend, seems an impossible and unnecessary task, even harmful in the hands of the laity who have received no training."

In March 1833, about 18 months after the publication of Hartmann's ***Therapeutics***, Hahnemann left no doubt as to his uncompromising position about the necessity of keeping homeopathy pure in the preface of the 5th edition of the ***Organon***. He wrote: "Homeopathy is a perfectly simple system of medicine remaining always fixed in its principles as in its practice, which, like the doctrine whereon it is based, if rightly apprehended, will be found to be so exclusive (and *only in that way* serviceable) that as the doctrine must be accepted in its purity, so it must be purely practiced, and all backward straying to the pernicious routine of the old school (whose opposite it is, as day to night) is totally inadmissible, otherwise it ceases to deserve the honourable name of homeopathy."

"That some misguided physicians who would wish to be considered homeopathists, engraft some, to them more familiar, allopathic malpractices upon their nominally homeopathic treatment, is owing to ignorance of the doctrine, laziness, contempt for the suffering humanity, and ridiculous conceit; and, besides showing unpardonable negligence in searching for *the best* homeopathic specific for each case of disease, has often a base love of gain and other sordid motives for its spring/and for its results? that they cannot cure all important and serious diseases (which pure and careful homeopathy can) and that they send many of their patients to that place whence no one returns, whilst the friends console themselves with the reflection that everything (including every hurtful allopathic process!) has been done for the departed."

Hahnemann intended that his reprimand of Hartmann be seen as a warning to prevent future misrepresentations of our strict and exacting method when an attempt is made to make the practice of homeopathy more accessible at the expense of the patient's welfare. Since that time, a great number of clinical guides have been published, most of them neglecting Hahnemann's warning by being gross misrepresentations of our science. However a small number of clinical guides have been presented which were within the realms of pure homeopathy. Jahr's ***Clinical Guide*** was one of the first ones to provide a better differential materia medica. Then we saw the appearance of Boenninghausen's ***Therapeutics of Intermittent Fevers*** and later ***Treatment of Hooping Cough***. Here in America some true classics were published such as Bell's ***Diarrhea***, Guernsey's ***Obstetrics***, Minton's ***Uterine Therapeutics***, Allen's ***Therapeutics of Fever***, Yingling's ***Accoucheur's Emergency Manual***,

Nash's ***Leaders in Respiratory Organs***, Pulford's ***Pneumonia***, Robert's ***Rheumatic Remedies***, and in England, Tyler's ***Pointers***.

Dr. Thomas Kruzel is now presenting to the profession in this ***Homeopathic Emergency Guide*** a very practical and reliable guide to assist the practitioner of homeopathy in those cases of acute crisis when "time is short and judgement difficult." Every conscientious practitioner of homeopathy will find this guide a quick and valuable reference. If this guide is used with the understanding of the absolute necessity to constantly individualize our cases it can only increase our clinical success. Generalization and routinist thinking will inevitably spell failure, not for homeopathy or the Law of Similars, but for the practitioner and unfortunately, for his/her patient. Since Hahnemann, the keys to success have always been first to make a thorough and skillful examination of the sick and then to carefully choose the remedy which is the most similar to the totality of the characteristic symptoms of the patient.

Often at the bedside of the sick in acute crises the symptoms may appear deficient, especially in cases presenting with a lowered state of consciousness. One will have then to patiently and carefully examine the sick person and question the attendants until clues indicating the simillimum are discovered. Lippe, the prince of prescribers, was so right when he said that "patients do not often give the symptoms as we would wish them to give and we have then to apply our individual judgement to find by interrogation what the real, true symptoms of the sick are. But we must never rest till we obtain a clear conception of the case before us."

Some imperfections may be found in this work like in any other work of this type. As this manual represents the cumulative experience of the profession it will continue to mature with time. Additions must be constantly entered, refinements and corrections made to the point of precision, and differentiation pushed further. When future editions of this manual become warranted the author will judiciously add that cumulative experience and further complete this already very reliable manual.

I recommend this practical and valuable manual coming from Dr. Thomas Kruzel, an able and honest worker of homeopathy.

Andre Saine, N.D., D.H.A.N.P.
August 1992

Introduction

While a student at the National College of Naturopathic Medicine in Portland, Oregon, studying homeopathy, I found that there was a difference between the remedy presentations studied in the classroom and what I saw clinically. Unless a remedy picture was made very clear by the patient or it could be narrowed down by repertorising, it was often difficult to arrive at the prescription without prolonged analysis. In acute cases or in a busy clinical practice, time is often a precious commodity. Thus, it became necessary for me to study the remedies according to condition, comparing those most commonly prescribed. This work, then, is a continuance of that study, and its preparation has greatly enhanced my own homeopathic prescribing skills.

This book is not meant to replace study of the homeopathic materia medica, good case taking or repertorising skills. Nor should it take the place of a thorough case analysis in chronic disease prescribing. In order to use this book more effectively, you must be well versed in these areas. As every homeopath is aware, homeopathy is a life-long study.

Used in conjunction with books such as ***Homeopathic Medicine at Home*** by Maesimund Panos and Jane Heimlich, or Dana Ullman and Stephen Cummings' excellent book ***Everybody's Guide to Homeopathic Medicine***, the ***The Homeopathic Emergency Guide*** fills a need for those people who have not quite mastered the art of repetorisation and case analysis. I continue to encourage many of my patients, especially those with families, to purchase home remedy kits and the books mentioned so that they can treat themselves and their loved ones at home.

This is also written for the clinician who possesses a strong background and desires a quick reference in an office, emergency or inpatient setting. Further, it is hoped that those physicians who do not utilize homeopathy as much as they would like will be able to do so with the prescribers' aid.

So how does one use this work? The conditions are listed in alphabetical order as are the remedies most often found to cure patients with these or similar conditions. In some instances a specific section may not be found for the condition but a combination of several will help with remedy selection. As an example, postpartum hemorrhage, which is blood loss following childbirth, can be consulted for bleeding between the periods, as it involves bleeding from the uterus. The section on hemorrhages may also be consulted in this case in addition to being used for other types of bleeding episodes.

Each section begins with a brief description of the disorder or condition along with some guidelines as to what constitutes a medical emergency and what necessitates a physician's evaluation. This is primarily for those who have no medical training and are unsure when the person needs to be referred to a doctor.

Numbers in parentheses following the remedies are taken from the corresponding rubric or rubrics in **Kent's Repertory**. They are provided to give the prescriber an idea of the remedies usefulness. Thus, under the **Hayfever—Allergies** section, the (3) following **Allium cepa** (All-c) is taken from the rubric **Nose Coryza, annual** (hayfever). This means that this particular remedy is often found to be useful in the treatment of hayfever. Under the same heading, **Arsenicum alb** (Ars alb) is followed by a (2). This means that this remedy also affects hayfever but not as often as **Allium cepa**. Roman type remedies such as **Lachesis** (Lach) also affect hayfever but not nearly as often as the others. If no numbers are present, there was no rubric consulted or the remedy was not listed in the one used. Remedies in parentheses which are found following symptoms mean that the remedy should also be considered if that symptom is present in the case.

Items in **boldface type** correspond to boldface type in the repertory or materia medica. This means that the symptom is almost always seen and affected by the remedies action. ***Italicized boldface type*** is used when the symptom is a keynote of the remedy or a symptom which is only seen with this remedy.

The symbols < (worse with) and > (better with) precede the remedy's modalities and are standard homeopathic notations familiar to all homeopaths worldwide. Modalities are special attributes which characterize the individual remedies. They are useful to the prescriber in that they help distinguish one remedy from another. As an example, the remedy Sulphur is better with lying still and worse with motion. This is noted as "> lying still and < motion" at the end of the remedies description. Rhus tox is better with motion and worse with lying still, as is noted by "> motion and < lying still." Comparison of these modalities helps to decide which remedy to give.

An attempt has been made to note modalities which are specific to the disease condition in order not to confuse them with other general conditions that the remedy may also cover. The student is cautioned not to exclude a remedy if all of these modalities are not present, but rather to base a prescription on the symptoms that are present in the case.

Some of the more common mental/emotional and general symptoms of the various remedies have been included. This does not mean that they need to be present during these conditions, but rather that they are often seen with them and may be part of the presentation.

Several of Dr. Stephen Messer's excellent flow charts are found at various places throughout the book. I have found them to be a very useful and valuable asset to prescribing, as well as an excellent learning tool. They can be used to help narrow your remedy selections before further study.

Lastly, I have included rubrics (symptoms) at the end of each section which I and others have found useful in prescribing. These are to help the practitioner decide between remedies when the picture is unclear. Rubrics (symptoms) are located under the section headings in repertories which list all the remedies that have been found to have that particular symptom. Thus **Nose Coryza, annual** (hayfever) is a rubric found on page 256 under the **Nose, Coryza** section of **Kent's Repertory**. Many of the remedies in the **Hayfever—Allergies** section of this book were taken from this rubric. The remedies under this section are far from complete, and I encourage each of you to compile your own as you go along.

What is the best way to use this book? For myself, I continue to use it the way I always have since my student clinic days, which is to take as thorough a case as I am able, including any observations and physical examination findings. Consultation with my repertory helps in narrowing the possible remedy choices. Once this is done, I consult the HMG to help in my selection of the simillimum. The simillimum is that remedy which best matches the presenting symptoms or disease state with which you are faced. Each of you, however, will develop your own style depending upon your level of experience and familiarity with homeopathy.

In the past few years, homeopathic medicine has continued to grow and gain acceptance. It has become one of the fastest-growing industries in Europe and is becoming more recognized as a viable alternative to conventional drug therapy. In addition, our health care system in the United States has become so large and costly that not only medical consumers, but government and industrial leaders are calling for alternatives. Homeopathy offers solutions to these problems as evidenced by its steady and continual growth.

In conclusion, I encourage you to make your own notes in the margins as you gain experience in order to add to the growing body of homeopathic knowledge. This work is far from complete and is more a reflection of my compiling skills than that of a prescriber. In light of this I welcome input, so this book can be updated and made more useful. It is my hope that however this work is utilized, it will be for the betterment of your patients and the advance of homeopathy.

Thomas A. Kruzel N.D.
May, 1992
Corbett, Oregon

Symbols Used In This Book

Bold Face Type	Symptom is Always Seen
Italicized	Keynote of the Remedy
>	Better With
<	Worse With
(3)	Remedy Often Indicated for the Condition
(2)	Remedy Occassionally Indicated for the Condition
(Lach)	Remedy With Same Symptom to Also Consider
Rubric	Sections in the repertory which list patient symptoms and the corresponding remedies.

ABDOMINAL INFLAMMATION

Abdominal pain and **inflammation** present difficulties in diagnosis for even the most experienced physicians because there are many conditions that cause it. The problem may range from entrapment of gas due to constipation, perforation of the bowel which results in severe inflammation, and sepsis which may result in death. Therefore, any acute onset of abdominal pain should be considered a medical emergency and a physician needs to be consulted as soon as possible.

In my experience, homeopathic medicine works quite well in the treatment of an acute abdomen, often averting the need for surgery in a number of cases. Giving the medicine prior to referral to the emergency room, they were generally doing better by the time they arrived, resulting in observation rather than surgery.

Prescriptions, however, are always made with caution. Consideration is given as to possible outcomes if homeopathic treatment is undertaken and changes in symptom patterns which may require a second prescription. Therefore, frequent follow-up to monitor the patient's condition is a must.

GASTRITIS, DIARRHEA

Aloe

Pain around navel; < pressure; **abdomen feels full**, **heavy**, hot; bloated; flatulence, **pulsation in rectum after eating**; nausea with headache; weak; feels as if diarrhea will come; much flatus pressing downward; **sensation of a plug between coccyx and pubes**, with urging; stool passes without effort, unnoticed, **burning in anus**, rectum; **much mucus and pain in rectum after stool**; averse to meat; longs for juicy things; stool escapes with flatus or with urinating; internal sensation of heat; **sense of insecurity in rectum**, when passing gas.

< heat; damp, summer	> cool, open air
< early AM; after dysentery	> cold applications
< stepping hard; evening	
< hot; dry weather	
< after eating; drinking	

Arsenicum alb (3)

Nausea; retching; vomiting after eating or drinking; **cannot bear the sight or smell of food** (Colch); **great thirst**, **drinks much**, **but a little at a time**; **burning pains**; anxiety in pit of stomach; vomits blood; bile; green mucus; brown-black mixed with blood; stomach extremely irritable, seems raw; dyspepsia from vinegar, acids, ice cream, ice water, tobacco; everything seems to lodge in esophagus; fear, dyspnea with gastralgia; **small**, **offensive**, **dark stools with much prostration**; stool **< night**; **eating**; **drinking**; **cadaveric odor**; **very restless**, **chilly**, **craves ice water which distressed stomach**; foul, rice water stools; **restless**; food poisoning; gradual weight loss.

< cold, **ice**, **drinks**, **food**, air	**> hot**, **applications**, **food**
< periodically; **midnight**; **after 2 AM**	> hot drinks; sweating
< vegetables; **drinking**	> motion; **elevating head**
< eruptions; suppressed, undeveloped	> sitting erect; company
< exertion; tobacco; lying on part	
< seashore; right side	

Chamomilla (2)

Distended abdomen; gripping pain in region of navel, pain in small of back; bilious vomiting; regurgitation of food; averse to warm drinks; nausea after coffee; pressive gastralgia as from a stone (Abies n, Bry); foul eructations; hot, **green**, watery, fetid, **slimy** stool, with colic; chopped white and yellow mucus; anus sore; dentition diarrhea; colic goes upward; **lienteric stools**; hot and thirsty or hot sweat with the pain; **ugly**, **cross**, **uncivil**; **quarrelsome**; oversensitive; intolerance of pain; **thirsty**; night sweats.

< anger; **night**; **dentition**	**> being carried**, **held**
< cold, air, damp, wind	> mild weather; heat
< taking cold; **coffee**, alcohol	> sweating; cold applications
	> warm, wet weather

China

Tender, cold stomach; vomits undigested food; sensation of a weight after eating; hungry without an appetite; pains dart crosswise in hypochondrium; milk aggravates; **belches** bitter fluid or regurgitation of food **gives no relief**; bloatedness > movement; **flatulence**, with colic > bending double (Coloc); **tympanic abdomen**; internal coldness of stomach and abdomen; right hypochondrial pain; undigested stool; frothy; yellow; **painless** stool, < night; after meals, **fruit**; milk, beer; stool very weakening; much flatulence; **lienteric stool; bloody stool**; **drenching sweats at night**; **debility**; apathetic; indifferent; **thirsty**; chilly.

< vital losses; **touch**; noise
< periodically, alternate days
< cold; drafts; wind
< open air; mental exertion
< eating; fruit; milk
< bending over

> hard pressure
> loose clothes
> bending over double
> open air, warmth

Colocynthis (2)

Drawing pain; sensation as if something would not yield in stomach; agonizing; cutting pain in abdomen; **causes patient to bend over double**; presses on abdomen; sensation as if stones were being ground together in abdomen, and would burst; bruised feeling of intestines; colic with cramps in calves; cutting pain in abdomen especially after anger; paroxysms of pain accompanied by agitation and a chill over cheeks; ascending from hypogastrium; pain in small spot below navel; **dysenteric stool renewed each time by least food or drink**; **jelly-like stools**; musty odor; **sudden**, **violent cramping**; **grasping**; **clutching or radiating abdominal pains double patient up > hard pressure**; cutting pain in bowels, pressure > at first then <: yellow, frothy, watery, sourish stools; pain under right scapula; extremely irritable; gets angry with being questioned; thirsty.

< emotions; **vexation**
< chagrin; anger; lying on painless side

> hard pressure; coffee
> heat; rest
> gentle motion

< night, in bed; drafts
< taking cold

> after stool; flatus
> doubling up
> lying with head bent forward

Croton tig

Burning in esophagus; copious, watery stools, with much urging; **always forcibly shot out**; with gurgling in intestines; constant urging to stool, followed by sudden evacuations with flatus; **swashing/ gurgling sensation in intestines**; alternating diarrheas and **skin eruptions**; **projectile stool**; **profuse**, **gushing yellow watery stool < drinking**; condition often alternates with skin eruptions or asthma; cholera infantum; pain in abdomen from diarrhea which is < touch; **sense of fullness in rectum**; diarrhea comes and goes with chilliness of the back and a certain amount of facial heat; often has weakness from passing stool.

< drinking; eating
< washing; motion
< receding eruptions
< during summer
< touch; AM and PM

> sleep

Dulcamara

Vomiting of white, tenacious mucus or greenish-yellow and slimy mucus; **averse to food**; **burning thirst for cold drinks**; heartburn; nausea with desire for stool; **chilliness during vomiting**; colic from cold; **cutting pain about navel**; stool green, watery, slimy, bloody, **mucus**, especially in summer when weather turns cold, from **damp**, **cold weather**; repelled eruptions; sour, watery stools, < night; thirsty, **chilly**; shooting pains in abdomen; rumbling with nausea, eructation and vertigo; green frothy diarrhea expelled with much force; stool pains unnoticed ; nausea with inability to vomit.

< while hot; sudden temperature changes
< uncovering; **cold wet**, feet, ground, cellars; beds
< being chilled; sweat; eruptions
< autumn; night; rest; injuries
< before storms

> moving about
> external warmth
> rest; open air

Elaterium

Nausea, eructations, vomiting, with great weakness; sense of enlargement of nasopharynx; gripping bowel pains or may be painless; violent vomiting; stools are **watery**, **copious**, **forceful**; **squirting diarrhea**; frothy; olive green, with sharp cutting in abdomen, may have an empty sensation; yawns all through the chill < exposure to damp ground; for use with true cholera.

Ferrum met

Voracious appetite or an absolute loss of appetite; loathing of sour things; attempts to eat bring on diarrhea; **spits up food by the mouthful** (Phos), eructation of food after eating, without nausea; nausea and vomiting after eating; **vomits immediately after eating**, **after midnight**; **intolerance of eggs**; heat and burning in stomach; distension and pressure after meals; soreness of abdominal walls; stools undigested; at night, while eating, drinking, are painless; ineffectual urging; averse to meat; painless lienteric diarrhea; diarrhea alternates with constipation; **chilly**; irritable; **intolerance of slightest noises**; sensitive; excitable.

< night; emotions; drinking
< violent exertion; eating
< sweating; loss of fluid
< eggs; heat and cold
< sudden motions; raising arms
aggravated at midnight
< washing

> gentle motion
> slight bleeding
> leaning head on something
> walking slowly about

Gambogia

Great irritability of stomach; feeling of coldness at edge of teeth; burning; smarting; dryness of tongue and throat; stomach pains after eating; epigastric tenderness; pain and distension of abdomen from flatulence, after stool; **rumbling and rolling**; dysentery; diarrhea with **sudden and forcible ejection** of bilious stool; **tenesmus after, with burning in anus**; ileo-cecal region tender to pressure; profuse, watery diarrhea, similar to Croton, in hot weather, in elderly; coccyx pain; **thin stool comes in prolonged gushes**; some thirst; head feels heavy.

< after stool
< motion in open air
< towards evening, at night

Gratiola

Pressure on epigastrium after a meal, as if a stone; which moves back and forth; paroxysms of wanting to vomit < with eructations; vertigo during and after meals; hunger and empty feeling after meals; dyspepsia with much distension of stomach; cramps, colic after supper, and during night; with swelling of abdomen and constipation; nausea, with cold in abdomen; diarrhea of **green**; **frothy** water; followed by anal burning; **forcibly evacuated without pain**; constipation with gouty acidity; rectum constricted; sensation as if cold water or a loose, heavy load in stomach; patient relieved after evacuation (Gamb); hypochondriasis; weak will; some thirst.

< eating; motion; summer
< coffee; dinner
< drinking too much water

Iris

Burning of whole alimentary canal; **vomiting**; **sour**, bloody, **biliary**; nausea; **deficient appetite**; cutting abdominal pain; sore liver; flatulent colic; diarrhea, **watery** stools with **burning at anus**, and through intestinal canal; periodical night diarrhea; with pain and green discharges; **constipation**; **pancreatitis**; headache and/ or nausea with diarrhea; urging to stool and profuse urination with periodic visual disturbances; burning not > with cold water; eyes and skin may be yellow; nausea or sick headache brought on by **eating anything sweet**.

< periodically, weekly, 2–3 AM	> gentle motion
< spring and fall; after midnight	
< mental exhaustion; hot weather	
< rest	> bending forward (colic)

Jatropha

Hiccough, followed by copious vomiting; nausea and vomiting brought on by drinking, with acrid feeling from throat; great thirst;

very easy vomiting; heat and burning in stomach, with crampy, constrictive pain in epigastrium; distended abdomen, with gurgling; pain in hypochondria; pain in liver and under right scapula to shoulder; sudden; profuse, rice water like stools; **forced discharge of diarrhea**; with **loud gurgling-like water coming out of a large hole**, **like a torrent**, associated with coldness, cramps, nausea and vomiting; **coldness** of whole body; violent cramps; stool > in AM; rumbling in abdomen with colic > walking in open air; not < by a loose stool.

< covering; morning; summer — > hands in cold water
< touch; pressure

Mercurius cor (2)

Bloated abdomen, painful to touch; bruised sensation; painful cecal region and transverse colon; incessant green, bilious vomiting; very sensitive epigastrium; dysentery; **tenesmus**, not > with stool; incessant; stool hot, **bloody**, **slimy**, offensive, with cutting pains and **shreds of mucous membranes**; gastritis; epigastric cramps; continuous urging to stool and urinate; **a never get done feeling** when passing stool; painful flatulence; violent thirst; chilly after stool; much perspiration; delirious, stupor, anxious; restless.

< after, **urinating**, **stool**, swallowing — > resting
< night; cold; autumn
< hot days; cool nights; acids

Mercurius (2)

Stomach sensitive to touch; putrid eructations; **intense thirst for cold drinks**; weak digestion with **continuous hunger**; violent vomiting with convulsive movements; burning; violent pain; sharp, constrictive pain in precordial region; violent empty eructations; painful sensitiveness of abdomen, < every movement; violent colic with diarrhea; cutting and lancinating pains; painful contractions primarily at night or cool of evening; abdominal pains > with lying down; sensation as if intestines were loose; acrid; **bloody**, knotty, viscid, pus, stools; complains before and during stool of pains; pain without stool; greenish; **slimy stools**, **< night**; **never get done feeling**; **thirsty**; chilly; weary of life; mistrustful; weakened, slow to answer.

< **night**; air; **sweating**	> moderate temperatures
< **lying on right side**; **drafts** to head	> bed rest
< **heated**; weather changes; cold	
< heat and cold; wet feet; firelight	
< touch	

Nux vomica (2)

Sour taste; **nausea in the AM, after eating**; **weight and pain in stomach, < eating, some time after**; sour, bitter eructations; **nausea and vomiting**; with much retching; **region of stomach very sensitive to pressure** (Ars, Bry); bloated epigastrium, with pressure as if a stone, **several hours after eating**; ravenous hunger, especially about a day before an attack of dyspepsia; dyspepsia from coffee; wants to vomit but cannot, difficult to belch; **abdomen feels bruised, sore** (Apis, Sulph); flatulent distension, with spasmodic colic; colic from uncovering; constipation, **with frequent, ineffectual urging**; **feels as if some remains**; irregular, peristaltic action; **ineffectual desire with passing of small quantities**; absence of all desire for defecation is a contraindication (Boericke); alternate constipation and diarrhea, after abuse of purgatives; diarrhea after over indulgence, > AM; dysentery; stools **relieve pains for a time**; **constant uneasiness in rectum**; diarrhea, with jaundice; heartburn; waterbrash; nausea > if they can vomit; gastric pains travel to back, chest; sensation as if a band around waist; < clothing around waist; **soreness of bowels, < coughing, stepping**; chill with thirst and heat with no thirst; **irritable**; **sensitive**; **sullen**; **impatient**; **violent**; cannot sleep after 3 AM; thirsty; **chilly**.

< **early AM**; **uncovering**	> **free discharges**; naps
< **cold**; **open air**, drafts, wind	> resting; wrapping head
< **high living**; **coffee**, alcohol, purgatives	> hot drinks; evenings
< sedentary habits; overeating	> moist air; milk
< mental, exertion, fatigue, vexation	> strong pressure
< disturbed sleep; dry cold weather	
< **slightest causes**, **pressure**, noise, odor	
< clothes about waist; touch	

Phosphoric acid

Craves juicy things; sour eructations; nausea; **symptoms occur after sour food and drink**; pressure as if a weight in stomach, with sleepiness after eating; **thirst for cold milk**, distended abdomen with fermentation; **aching in umbilical region**; loud rumbling; diarrhea, **white**, watery; involuntary; **painless** with much flatus; is not especially exhausting; diarrhea in weakly, delicate children; **weak or debilitated**, with free secretions; **stools lienteric**; **sleepy during the day** but awake at night; **apathetic**, **indifferent**; effects of grief, emotional shock; **chilly**.

< debility; **loss of fluids**, fatigue
< fevers; convalescence
< emotions; grief, shock, homesickness
< drafts; cold; music; talking
< being talked to

> warmth; short sleep
> stool

Podophyllum

Hot, sour, belching; nausea, vomiting; thirst for large quantities of cold water; vomits hot, frothy mucus; heartburn; gagging or empty retching; vomits milk; distended abdomen; heat and emptiness in abdomen; **sensation of weakness or sinking**; lies comfortably only on stomach; region of liver painful, **> rubbing part**; rumbling and shifting of flatus in ascending colon; **early AM diarrhea**, **during teething**; **with hot**, **glowing cheeks** while bathed; diarrhea in hot weather after acid fruits; green; watery, **fetid**, **profuse**, **projectile**, gushing; **rectal prolapse** before or during stool; alternating constipation and diarrhea (Ant c, Nux v); gastroenteritis with colic and bilious vomiting; weak, empty, sick feeling in stomach; **painless diarrhea**, summer diarrhea; whining, rolls head; depressed; bad breath; thirsty for large amounts of cold water (Bry).

< early AM; eating; hot weather
< dentition; drinking; motion

> stroking liver
> lying on abdomen

Rheum

Sour diarrheas; **whole child smells sour**; desires various kinds of food but soon tires of them; throbbing in pit of stomach; feels full; nausea, as if proceeding from stomach, with colic; fullness and pressure in stomach; colicky pain around navel; colic when uncovering; distended abdomen with tension; cutting in abdomen which force a curving of the body, often shortly after a meal, < standing; colic, < uncovering, > stool; unsuccessful urge to urinate before stool; **stools smell sour**, pasty, with shivering and tenesmus and burning in anus; urgent and frequent desire to evacuate without any result, < by movement, walking; liquor, slimy stools with pale face, ptyalism; child draws legs up; colic, > doubling up, < uncovering; indifference, impatient, vehement; restless, with desire to weep.

< dentition; eating	> warmth; wrapping up
< summer; nursing women	> lying doubled up
< uncovering; moving about	

Silicea (2)

Disgust for meat, **warm food**; swallowing food easily gets into posterior nares; want of appetite, excessive thirst; sour eructations after eating (Calc, Sep); pit of stomach painful to pressure; vomits after drinking (Ars, Verat);nausea, every AM, with pain in head, eyes, on turning eyes or followed by vomiting of bitter water; water-brash, sometimes with shuttering; continuous nausea, vomiting; burning sensation in pit of stomach; pressure in stomach; sometimes after every meal; painful cold or pain feeling in abdomen > external heat; hard, bloated; much rumbling in bowels; shooting pain in hypochondria, especially left side; pains < touch, walking, lying on right side; aching of abdomen, especially after a meal; **stool comes down with difficulty**; **partly expelled**, **then recedes**; diarrhea of cadaverous odor; difficult expulsion of flatus; soft stools expelled with difficulty; **foul foot sweats**; **chilly**; **very sensitive**; **ill effects of vaccination**; **suppurative processes**; **thirsty**.

< cold, **air**; **drafts**, damp	**> warm**, **wraps to head**
< uncovering; bathing	> becoming warm
< change of moon; night; alcohol	> profuse urination

< mental exertion;checked sweat
Sensitive to excitement, noise, light, jarring
< lying down, on left side
< thunderstorms

> wet or humid weather

Veratrum alb (2)

Voracious appetite; **thirst for cold water**; **is vomited as soon as swallowed**; averse to warm food; **copious nausea and vomiting**; **aggravated by drinking and least motion**; anguish in pit of stomach; great weakness after vomiting; gastric irritability with **chronic** vomiting of food; violent nausea which frequently almost induces syncope; violent vomiting with great weakness; exhaustion; wants to lie down; coldness of hands; shuddering of body with general heat; followed by heat in hands; excessive sensitivity in region of stomach; pain comes some minutes after eating, not > with pressure; burning pains, **inflammation** of stomach; sinking, empty, **cold feeling** in abdomen; abdominal pain before stool; nocturnal abdominal pains, with sleeplessness; pain throughout abdomen as if from hot coals; griping, twisting colic, > after stool; abdomen hard, distended; **stools large**, **with much straining until exhausted**, **with cold sweat**; very painful diarrhea, water, **copious**, **and forcible evacuated** followed by prostration; watery diarrhea, < motion; rice water stools, cholera; loose blackish, sanguineous, green, brown stools; burning in anus during stool; **sullen indifference**; frenzy of excitement; loquacity; deadly anguish; cannot bear to be left alone; but refuses to talk; **chilly**; **thirsty**; **skin cold** , blue.

< raising up; motion
< cold; lying on back
< puerperal states
< night; weather changes

> rubbing; eating
> lying with head low
> walking; warmth

PANCREATITIS

Conium (2)

Severe aching in and around liver; chronic jaundice; pains in right hypochondrium; sensitive; bruised, swollen, knife like pains; sensation as if a band around abdomen; lancinating pains in left hypochondria; even in AM in bed with oppression; stitching pain in spleen; spasmodic colic; offensive eructations with griping and heat, heartburn; pressure in epigastrium 2 to 3 hours after eating; painless diarrhea, stool may feel cold when passed.

< seeing moving objects; **alcohol**	> letting part hang down
< raising arms; after exertion	> fasting; in dark
< injury; night; cold	> motion; pressure
< lying; with head low	
< at rest	

Iodum (2)

Pancreatic disease; enlarged mesenteric glands; cutting abdominal pains; liver and spleen enlarged and sore; abdominal pains which return after every meal; ravenous hunger which relieves the pain; violent colic; cramp-like pains; trembling in abdomen, from pit of stomach to periphery, with much heat; restlessness, patient > from moving about.

< heat; **room**, air; wraps	**> cold**, **air**, bathing
< exertion; fasting; night; rest	> motion; eating
< when quiet; right side	> open air

Iris (2)—See above

Spongia (3)

Abdomen hard and tight; spasms of abdomen; viscera drawn up against diaphragm; pain left side; digging; choking > discharge of wind; heat in abdomen; fine stretching externally in abdomen; sensation as if something were moving; excessive thirst; **great hunger**; cannot stand tight clothes around abdomen (Lach, Nux v).

< dry; **cold**, wind	> lying with head low
< raised from sleep	> eating a little
< raising arms	> descending
< before 12 PM; ascending	

APPENDICITIS

Bryonia (3)

Burning pains; **stitches**; **< pressure**; **coughing**; **breathing**; tenderness of abdominal walls; tractive pains in hypochondrium extending to stomach and back, in the AM, after dinner, sometimes with vomiting; hard swelling in hypochondria and umbilical region; tearing in stomach, from hips to pit of stomach; **thirsty**; **for cold drinks**; right side; **averse to motion**.

< motion; **least**, **rising up**; **cough**	**> pressure**, **lying on painful part**
< dry; heat; cold	**> cool**; **open air**; **quiet**
< becoming hot; **hot room**, **weather**	> cloudy, damp days
< drinking while hot; touch	> drawing knees up
< vexation; early AM	> heat to inflamed part

Iris—See above

Mercurius cor (3)—See above

Phosphorus (3)

Feels cold; sharp, cutting pains; **weak**, **empty**, **gone feeling** felt in abdomen; pancreatic disease; abdomen hard, distended, especially after a meal; pain < lying on right side; painful pulsation in right hypochondrium; shooting pains sometimes with pallid face, shivering, headache; inflammation of intestines; intussusception; pressure outward against side of abdomen; flatulent colic; low spirits; easily vexed; fear of being alone; **desires cold drinks**, restless; fidgety; **suddenness of onset**.

< lying on left or painful side; **back**	> eating; sleep; sitting up;
< slightest causes; talking **emotions**	> rubbing
< odors; light; touch	> cold, food, water to face
< cold; **hands**, open air	> in dark; being touched

< warm ingesta; weather changes
< wind, cold; thunderstorms
< AM and PM; mental fatigue

Silicea (3)—See above

Symptoms in Kent's Repertory	**Page**
Abdomen, Clothing sensitive to	541
Abdomen, Diarrhea, sensation of	543
Abdomen, Distended, eating after	545
Abdomen, Passing flatus, ameliorates	545
Abdomen, Painful, flatus, ameliorates	545
Abdomen, Dropsy	546
Abdomen, Enlarged	546
Abdomen, Gurgling	550
Abdomen, Hard	550
Abdomen, Inflammation	552
Abdomen, Pain, must bend double	556
Abdomen, Pain, lying on abdomen ameliorates	558
Abdomen, Pain, pressure aggravates	559
Abdomen, Rumbling	601
Stomach, Eructations ameliorate	490
Stomach, Nausea, food thought of	507
Stomach, Nausea, food looking at	507
Stomach, Nausea, food smell of	507
Stomach, Vomiting violent	535

ABSCESSES/BOILS /CARBUNCLES

An abscess is a localized collection of pus caused by the disintegration of the surrounding tissues. A boil is caused by a breakdown in the skin's defense mechanism which allows bacteria to invade the hair follicles causing inflammation. It is usually well circumscribed and characterized by a central core of pus and blood. A carbuncle is an inflammation of the subcutaneous tissue which terminates in the sloughing and discharge of large amounts of decayed tissue and pus through one or several openings. It is almost always accompanied by intense swelling, fever and complaints of feeling ill.

These conditions are characterized by the formation and discharge of pus and dead tissue, which always attempt to drain outward. This is the body's way of keeping the infection from spreading inward to the more vital organs. Once the discharge has begun, it should not be disrupted. As long as the site of the discharge is kept clean, the infection will heal from its deeper layers.

Sepsis or blood poisoning is always a possibility even with drainage, due to the weakened immune system which may be incapable of fighting off the infection. Therefore, the person should be monitored as a sharp rise in temperature may indicate that the infection has gone deeper.

Any person with an abscess, carbuncle or boil that is not resolving or is slow to heal, or with a deficient immune system due to another disease, should be seen by a physician so that complications can be avoided.

Anthracinum (3)

Burning and **induration**, abscess formation which is **swollen**, **burning** (Ars, Tar c) and tends to ulcerate; **black** and **blue** discoloration blisters (Lach, Tar c); **boils**, **succession of boils**; glands are swollen, accompanied by severe pain; thick, black hemorrhages, **blood does not coagulate**; sloughing of skin; septicemia; insect stings; patient may be restless or exhausted and near collapse; crusty, oozing eruptions or dry skin which itches; foul-smelling discharges; tendency to gangrene.

Arsenicum alb (3)

Skin is **dry**, **rough**, **scaling**, **burning** and itching; ulcerations with offensive discharges or wounds which become infected, poisoned; discharges are **putrid** which tend to become necrotic with **bleeding**, **burning** pains but the patient feels **cold**, is **< cold**, **cold drafts** and **> warmth**, pains become < the colder the person becomes; skin feels **cold** and **dry**; bluish or reddish spots on skin; painful black pustules (Anth, Lach); eruption of small red pimples which increase in size and form into ulcerations, may appear scruffy (Psor); pustules filled with blood; ulcerations with raised, hard edges and a blue-black base surrounded by a red discoloration; tendency to gangrene (Anth); patients are restless, fearful and full of anxiety; **thirsty**; **chilly**.

< after midnight, **night**	**> heat**; **motion**
< cold, **cold drinks**	

Carbolic acid (1)

Swelling and roughness of skin; blue—violet color of skin which has an **offensive odor**; **burning**, itching of the skin which is > rubbing, rubbing may be followed by burning (Kreos); eruption of fine vesicles; burns which ulcerate; discharges are foul-smelling; consider with sepsis and extreme prostration from burns, especially if no response to Veratrum album.

Hepar sulph (3)

Abscesses and ulcerations which are ***very sensitive to touch***, **cold**, **patient wants them covered**, **warm**; ulcerations bleed easily, smell like old cheese; pains are **sticking**, stinging and burning or itching; ulcerations **surrounded by small pimples**; skin is dry and chapped with cracks on hands and feet (Caust, Petr); foul, moist eruptions in folds of skin (Graph), **with easy suppuration**; very sensitive cold sores; considered useful in boils in lower potencies given frequently; cellulitis due to streptococcus (Rhus t) in early stages to halt the progress; patient is **very irritable** and may not let you do examination or will react violently to touch of lesion; thirsty; **chilly**.

< dry, cold wind	**> warmth**
< cold; touch	> wrapping up affected site

Lachesis (3)

Boils, carbuncles, ulcerations that have a **bluish-purple appearance**; dissecting wounds with surrounding bluish-purple discoloration which is very sensitive to touch (Hepar) and warmth; blisters which are dark with discharges of blue-black blood (Anthr, Ars); bed sores with black edges; purpura with prostration (Ars); scars which become red, painful, break open and bleed, **patient is > with discharges**; bed sores and ulcerations of legs and back (Ars); patients will be beside themselves with anxiety until abscess is lanced or breaks open (see Myristica); is weak, exhausted.

< after sleep, mornings	**> discharges, bleeding**
< warmth	

Mercurius (3)

Irregular-shaped ulcerations, abscesses, boils that have a lardaceous base and tend to spread; **moist eruptions**; pimples around main eruptions; vesicles which discharge a milky or opaque fluid which may have an odor like stale fish and/or streaks of blood; **itching** and **burning** of the skin; skin rash is red, rough and may be accompanied by a fever, rash may extend beyond initial site to cover the whole body and discharge large amounts of fluid; patient is chilly but cannot stand extremes of temperature; chilly; **thirsty**; (consider Mezereum if a partial response to Merc).

< becoming heated	> rest
< heat and cold	
< night	

Pyrogen (2)

Septic states, septic fevers, those caused by dissecting wounds and abscesses (Anthr); intense pain and burning in the abscess (Anthr); small cuts which become swollen, inflamed; skin is pale, cold, ashen; ulcerations which are offensive, **foul-smelling** (Ars);

decubitus ulcers in the elderly which do not heal; patient cannot lie still but must constantly change position which ameliorates for a while (Ars); person is **loquacious** (Lach), speaking very rapidly; **sensitive** (Cham, Nux) and anxious (Acon, Ars); **red streaks extending** from abscess or wound, discharges which are of a **foul odor**; bed feels hard (Arn).

< cold, damp	> hot, hot bath
	> change of position

Rhus tox (2)

Itching, **burning** and **stinging** of the skin, may have a sensation of being stuck with hot needles; **vesicular eruptions** with oozing; red and swollen skin with a tendency toward scale formation; skin is **sensitive to cold air** (Hepar); patient feels stiff but wants to move about; **cellulitis**, vesicles form over abscesses; **sensation as if flesh has been torn loose from the bones**; abscess formation; patient may report that hot showers to skin feel orgasmic; thirsty; **chilly**.

< cold, damp	> warmth

Secale (2)

Burning sensation of the skin, ***patient wants parts uncovered even though skin feels cold to the touch;*** blue, mottled, dry, shriveled skin; **much aversion to heat**; sensation of formication under the skin; abscesses, boils and carbuncles which discharge a greenish pus and tend to bleed and heal slowly.

< heat, warm coverings	**> cold, uncovering**
< touch	
< loss of fluids	

Silicea (3)

One of the best medicines for boils, abscesses, carbuncles, ulcers and fistulas; suppurative and ulcerative conditions which are slow to heal; every injury ends in a discharge; **discharge is thin, irritating and offensive** which causes the surrounding skin to itch and may be sensitive to touch; painful scars; abscesses of joints, **abscesses which form after vaccination**; sensation of cold in the ulcer; itching < at night; lesions sensitive to cold and are > warmth; ingrown toenails

(Magnetic Polus Australius); crawling, itching of the skin; glands swell and are painless but itchy; abscesses of bones (Mez) which are sensitive to touch; fistula and abscesses which burrow and do not break open; lesions heal very slowly, with difficulty; aching, shooting, itching pains in the ulcerations; **chilly**; **thirsty**.

< cold, damp cold **> warmth, heat**
< touch

Tarentula cub (3)

Carbuncles which are burning, stinging, with a **purplish hue** (Anthr, Ars); abscesses which are very painful; lesion starts out small then swells and becomes inflamed, later becomes hard and **very painful**; lesion discharges from one or several sites a thick, fetid , greenish serous like exudate, may contain cellular matter; may form a large cavity, go on to gangrene and/ or sepsis; red track leads from wound (Lach); surface of lesion feels warm; patient may have a fever and chills with profuse sweating, condition may develop into an intermittent fever which is < evenings; diarrhea may also accompany the infection; chilly

< cold, cold drinks
< night

Consider:

Belladonna

Red, dry, **hot**, shining eruptions and **boils** which form quickly and spread; alternate **redness and paleness of the skin**, **very sensitive to touch** (Hepar); good early on to abort formation of abscesses, boils, carbuncles, cellulitis or whitlow; glandular abscesses; consider if a rapid, violent onset; often followed by Hepar as suppuration stage approaches.

Calcarea iod (3)

Ulcers, **accompanying varicose veins**; glandular swellings; tonsils which are enlarged and contain many crypts (Bar c); itching of skin which appears on different parts of the body, > scratching.

Calcarea sulph (3)

Suppurative processes, purulent discharges.

Myristica

Reported to hasten suppurations and shorten their duration; opens abscesses; considered the "homeopathic scalpel" as it acts similar to both Hepar and Silica and has been used rather than surgery to drain abscesses; antiseptic powers; anal fistula; suppurative otitis.

Sulphur (2)

Dryness of the skin with itching and roughness (Ars); **flaking** of the skin with itching, itching may be **> or < with scratching**, washing; fistulous ulcers or encysted swellings; induration or suppuration of glands; crops of boils or pimply eruptions which itch; **eruptions alternate with other complaints**; < heat.

Symptoms in Kent's Repertory	**Page**
Head, Abscess	107
Ear, Abscess	285
Nose, Abscess	324
Mouth, Abscess, gums	397
Teeth, Abscess, of roots	430
External Throat, abscess	471
Abdomen, Abscess, in walls	541
Rectum, Abscess	606
Chest, Abscess	822
Back, Abscess	884
Extremities, Abscess	952
Generalities, Abscesses	1343
Generalities, Cold, becoming, amel/agg.	1349
Generalities, Heated, becoming agg.	1367

ASTHMA

The term **asthma** is used generally to describe any disorder of impaired breathing involving a reversible airway obstruction. It often occurs secondarily to a variety of external stimuli such as smoke, changes in temperature, emotional upsets or exposure to specific allergens. It is also seen more commonly in children than adults, and a relationship to foods such as milk or wheat has been noted. A history of prior upper respiratory infection is also common.

Symptoms may range from mild to severe and include wheezing, rapid and labored breathing, cough, tightness in the chest, shortness of breath and increased mucus with expectoration.

"Attacks" of asthma quite often occur at night due to mucus buildup in the airways with lying down. Hypersensitivity reaction or foreign-body aspiration must be considered in younger children who develop a sudden onset of difficulty with breathing and have had no previous history. **Inflammation of the larynx**, called **epiglottitis**, is a potentially fatal condition and examination must be done with great care by a physician with knowledge of intubation procedures.

Most persons experiencing an asthma attack will exhibit varying degrees of distress until the cause has been eliminated or the body is able to restore the balance. A sudden worsening of the patient's respiratory distress or change in symptoms is a signal to the examiner that some type of intervention may be necessary and the person needs to see a physician.

Ammonium carb (2)

3 AM (Cupr); **marked oppression of breathing**; severe asthma; exhausted breathing; shortness of breath with marked wheezing, bronchial constriction, congestion; difficult expectoration; burning in chest; cough with palpitations; worse ascending; slow, labored, stertorous breathing; bubbling sounds, pulmonary edema; slimy

sputum with specks of blood; **weakness of heart**; aphonia, lacks reaction; **weak and drowsy**; chilly.

< cold, cloudy days	**> pressure**
< damp, open air	> eating
< 3–4 AM, motion	> lying on abdomen
< menses	> dry weather
< wet application	

Aralia racemosa

9–11 PM; **dry cough with first sleep**, **asthma on lying down at night**; **tickling or foreign-body sensation in throat**, strong cough, spasmodic cough; constriction of chest; rawness burning behind sternum; **frequent sneezing**; hay fever; least draft of air causes sneezing; **copious watery excoriating nasal discharge**; **salty acrid taste**; whistling breathing; drenching sweat during sleep.

< 11 PM, after a nap	> lying with head high
< drafts	> sitting up

Arsenicum alb (3)

11:30 to 2–3 AM—**very restless**, may alternate with prostration, burning in chest, **sips warm drinks**, **anxious**, association with skin eruptions (alternate) (Ars-i—if underlying pollen or hay fever); can't lie down, fear of suffocation; cough worse lying on back; scanty expectoration—**frothy**; **darting pain**, **upper portion of right lung**; wheezing respiration; dry cough; bloody sputum; cough alternately dry and loose, must sit up; cough worse drinking; **fear of death**; sudden onset; **air hunger**; thirsty for warm drinks; chilly.

< cold drinks, air	> hot applications, food, drink
< 11:30 to 3 AM	> motion
< exertion	> elevating head, sitting up
< yearly bouts	> company, sweating
congestion to head > cold	

Arsenicum iod (3)

Cough dry with little and difficult expectoration; hacking cough; **asthma associated with hay fever**; air hunger; short of breath; yellow/green foul expectoration; asthma of psoric persons; burning heat in chest; thirsty; chilly.

< dry, cold weather	> open air
< windy, foggy	
< exertion, in a room	
< apples, tobacco smoke	

Cuprum met (3)

3 AM (Am c); cough with gurgling sound, **better drinking cold water**; suffocative attacks; **spasm and constriction of chest**; spasmodic asthma alternates with spasmodic vomiting; dyspnea with uneasy sensation in epigastrium; angina with asthma; breathing worse with bending backward; loud rattle in chest; painful constriction of chest; severe spasmodic cough ending with patient becoming motionless and stiff or goes into convulsions; symptoms change suddenly in character; severe weakness with illness.

< anger, motion	> cold drinks
< suppressions	> pressure over heart
< hot weather, touch	
< vomiting, loss of sleep	
< raising arm	

Ipecac (3)

Constant constriction in chest, incessant or suffocating cough; violent cough with every breath; cough causes nausea, gagging, vomiting; **coughs till they are blue in the face**; croup, **hoarseness from a cold; rattle in chest without expectoration; painless hoarseness**; child becomes stiff, with blueness of their face; **especially indicated if associated with nausea and vomiting** and/or frothy stool; thirstless; chilly.

< warmth, damp	> open air
< overeating, in a room	
< heat and cold	
< periodically	
< moist warm wind	
< lying down	

Kali carb (3)

2–4 AM, better with sitting up; **ameliorated by leaning forward**; plump, pale, tired; very sensitive to cold; anxiety in stomach; heart palpitations; frequent **eczema on palms**; stitching; cutting pains; dryness of pharynx; much expectoration in AM and after eating; **worse right lower chest**; **whole chest sensitive**; cheesy-tasting sputum; coldness of chest; **difficulty swallowing** tough sputum; head cold leading to chest cold; averse to solitude; **puffiness of upper eyelids between eyebrows and lid may occur with excessive coughing**; thirst and thirstless; **chilly**.

< cold air, **weather**, drafts	> warmth
< 2–3 AM, winter	> sitting with elbows on knees
< lying on painful side	> open air
< left side	

Kali nit (3)

Violent excessive dyspnea, dry AM cough with chest pain and bloody expectoration; cough is short, dry; hacking; dyspnea so severe that breath cannot be held long enough to drink; chest feels constricted; sour-smelling; clotted, bloody sputum; **spasmodic croup**; right lung congestion; palpitations; e**xternal coldness and internal burning**.

< walking, cold, damp	> gentle motion
< eating veal	> drinking sips of water
< lying with head low	

Lachesis (2)

Sensation of suffocation on lying down, **especially if anything is around throat**; wants windows open; **feels they must take a deep breath**; cough is dry, suffocative fits; **breathing almost stops on falling asleep** (Grind); larynx is painful to touch; better with expectoration; sensation of a plug which moves up and down with short cough (Anac); thirsty; cold; loquacious, sleep into their aggravation.

< sleep, AM, heat	> open air, cold drinks
< warm drinks	> discharges, expectoration
< swallowing	> hard pressure, bathing

< slight touch, noise	> warm applications
< retarded discharges	
< cloudy weather	

Lobelia (3)

Dyspnea from constriction of chest, sensation of pressure or weight in chest better **rapid walking**; asthma attack with weakness felt in pit of stomach and preceded by **prickling all over**; senile emphysema; sits with elbows on knees; rattling in chest with difficult expectoration; weak pulse.

	> rapid waking
< after sleep, tobacco	> evening
< suppressions	> warmth
< slightest motion	> eating a little

Natrum sulph (2)

4–5 AM; **holds chest when coughing** (Bry); **asthma from cold, damp weather**; heavy cough with ropy greenish expectoration; **empty**, **all-gone feeling in the chest**; desires to take a deep long breath; pain through **left lower chest**; fresh cold brings on asthma attack (Dulc); constitutional remedy for **asthma in children**.

< damp weather, night air	> open air
< damp cellars	> change of position
< lifting, touch, pressure	> dry weather
< wind, light	> pressure
< late evening; music	

Pulsatilla (3)

Evenings; dry night cough leading to loosening up in AM; bland, thick mucus, yellow/green; marked shortness of breath; anxiety, especially in evening; better sitting up; **pressure upon chest**, **soreness**; urine emitted with cough (Caust); feels smothered when lying down; **thirstless**; **weepy**; discouraged, desires sympathy; **air hunger**; asthma from suppressions; **thirstless**.

< warm room, bed, clothes	> open air, uncovering
< warm air, suppressions	> erect posture
< evening, rest	> gentle motion,

< before menses
< lying on left side, painless side
< first motion
< rich foods, fats
< pregnancy

continued motion
> weeping

Sambucus (3)

Midnight, child awakens with laryngeal spasm or suffocation; marked profuse sweating and cyanosis; mucus obstructs; rapid onset; spasmodic croup; difficult expectoration; chest oppression with pressure in stomach and nausea; if nursing, child cannot breathe; **cannot expire** (Meph); whistling breathing, spasm of glottis; **dry burning heat during sleep but copious sweat on waking**; thirstless.

< dry, cold air
< cold drinks
< while heated
< head low
< sleep
< after eating fruit

> pressure over a sharp edge
> motion, wrapping up
> sitting up

Senega (2)

Dryness, with a scraping, raw pain in the chest which is < talking; voice is hoarse and unsteady, loss of voice with reading aloud; sputum production is profuse, thick and very difficult to expectorate, may be blood-streaked or albuminous in consistency; soreness of chest with coughing, burning in chest from coughing; cough often ends with sneezing; rattling of mucus in chest; consider using in older persons with asthmatic bronchitis, hydrothorax (Merc, Sulph) or pneumonia; thirsty.

< inhaling cold air
< touch, **rest**
< walking in open air

> bending head backwards
> perspiration

Silicea (3)

Profuse mucopurulent sputum; slow recovery from pneumonia; stitches in chest through to back; **violent cough when lying**

down with thick yellow lumpy expectoration; retching, shaking gagging cough; **very sensitive** to noise, pain or cold; emaciation; mentally, alert, physically weak; **sweat** is profuse on upper body; **ailments from suppressed foot sweats, immunizations**; **thirsty**, **chilly**.

< cold feet
< uncovering
< new moon, night
< mental exertion, alcohol
< noise, jarring
< excitement
< lying on left side

> warm wraps to head
> profuse urination
> wet, humid weather

Spongia (3)

Much dryness of air passages; **hoarseness**; **larynx dry**, **burning**, **constricted**; **dry**, **croupy**, **barking cough**; **croup worse during inspiration and before midnight;** respiration is short, panting, **difficult**; **sensation of a plug in larynx**; **cough better after eating or drinking**, especially warm; irrepressible cough from deep in chest; wheezing cough worse from cold air; oppression of chest with weakness and heat; blue lips; larynx painful from touch; grabs throat when swallowing.

< dry, cold wind
< awakened from sleep
< exertion, raising arms
< using voice

> lying with head low
> eating
> coughing and

Sulphur (3)

Oppression, burning in chest; **difficult respiration**, **wants windows open**; loose cough; heat in chest; **much rattling of mucus**; chest feels heavy; stitching pains shoot to back; **oppression as if a load on chest**; dyspnea during night better with sitting up; **pulse more rapid in AM than PM**; irregular breathing; violent cough, 2–3 incomplete bouts; red/brown spots over chest; sulphur constitution; **thirsty**; chilly.

< bathing, suppressions
< milk

> open air, motion
> warm applications

< heated in bed, exertion
< speaking, atmospheric changes
< 11 AM, full moon
< at rest

> sweating, dry heat
> drawing up affected limbs
> on right side

Consider:

Chamomilla

Consider in **children** who are irritable and attack comes on during or after anger or tantrum; also in adults when attacks come on from anger (Ars, Nux v), or if condition is ameliorated with chamomille tea.

Medorrhinum (2)

3–5 AM, oppressed breathing, incessant dry night cough, can't exhale.

Nux vomica (2)

Aggravated midnight and 4–5 AM: Nux-vom leads to Arsenicum.

Thuja (3)

3 AM, 3 PM, child's remedy for asthma.

< night, heat of bed
< cold damp air

> left side
> drawing up limbs

Croup triad: Trio of remedies which often follow one another for the treatment of coughs and croup.

Aconite (3), **Hepar** (2), **Spongia** (3).

Symptoms in Kent's Repertory	**Page**
Respiration, Asthmatic	763
Respiration, Asthmatic, midnight, after	764
Respiration, Asthmatic, in children	764
Respiration, Asthmatic, emotions, after	764
Respiration, Asthmatic, eruptions suppressed	765
Respiration, Asthmatic, hay asthma	765

BACK PAIN—LUMBAGO

Back pain may be caused by a number of conditions including arthritis, osteoporosis, facet syndrome, herniated or ruptured disk, fibrositis, ligament and muscular strain, bone cancer and malingering. Diagnosis of the exact cause may be difficult as patients tend to manifest different symptoms for the same "disease."

In general, localized pains are due to **fibrositis** or muscular inflammation, while diffuse aching (lumbago) pains are seen with degenerative conditions such as **arthritis** or **osteoporosis**. With sharper, radiating pains you need to consider **rupture** of the **intervertebral disk**, **fracture** or compression of the vertebrae.

Limitation of motion is found with all of the pains described due to reflex muscle spasm; but pain with coughing, sneezing or passing stool should alert you to a possible ruptured disk. Rupture of the intervertebral disk is very painful and can lead to changes in sensation, ability to move the arms or legs, as well as severe muscle spasm. Referral to a physician is in order, as prolongation of the disk protrusion makes the chances of complete recovery less likely.

Back pain often benefits from physical therapy, massage or spinal manipulation which facilitates the healing process. In my experience, homeopathic medicine is an excellent complementary therapy to these treatments.

Aesculus (3)

Muscle weakness with pain; **low back gives out**, cannot provide support; feels tired and weak; Lumbo—Sacral weakness extends to hips; needs arm of chair for support; **dull pain**; lameness of neck, aching between scapulae; feet turn under when walking; soles feel tired, are sore and swell; hands and feet swell, become red after washing, feel full; affinity for sacro-iliac joint injuries, weakness; thirstless; chilly.

< AM, on waking	> cool open air, bathing
< after stool; lying, stooping	> bleeding hemorrhoids
< urinating, walking	> kneeling; exertion
< standing	> short sitting

Cimicifuga (2)

Cervicals, especially occiput, C1, L4, L5 pain with cervical pain; spine very sensitive especially upper; **stiffness and contraction in neck and back**; rheumatic pains; crick in back; uneasy restless feeling in limbs; oversensitive; worse during pain (Nux-vom); pain at angle of scapula; aching in limbs; **muscle soreness**; thirsty; chilly.

< lying, sitting with use of psoas	> warm wraps
< with flexion of neck	> open air; pressure
< menses; emotions	> continued motion
< alcohol, night	> grasping things; eating
< cold, damp air	
< heat and cold	
< sitting	
< change of weather	

Colocynth (2)

Contraction of muscles; limbs drawn together, or upward; **cramp-like pain in hip**; left-sided sciatica; pain down right thigh; numbness with pain (Gnaphal); tension neck and shoulder blades; drawing pains; **weakness in small of back**, especially with headache; coxofemoral joint as if fastened with an iron clasp; **sudden severe cramping**; **screwing**; band-like or shooting sciatic pains; thirsty.

< emotions, vexation	**> hard pressure**
< anger	> coffee; heat
< lying on painless side	> gentle motion
< night in bed; drafts	> after stool or flatus
< taking cold	
< gentle touch	

Gnaphalium

Chronic lumbar ache, **numbness** in lower back and weight in pelvis; burning pains alternating with numbness, weakness; usually right-sided; **intense pain along sciatic nerve alternates with numbness** (Coloc); better drawing up limbs; sciatica; < lying down; anterior crural neuralgia (Staph), cramps in calves and legs while in bed.

< motion, lying
< cold damp

> flexing limbs
> sitting

Kali bic (2)

Disks; wandering pains joint to joint (Kali s, Puls); **severe pain in small spots** (Oxalic ac); aching pain at night with lying; better in AM with motion; pain in sacrum with sitting up; pain in coccyx from rising and first sitting down; **cutting pains through loins**; pains extend up and down; bones feel sore and bruised; pain, swelling; stiffness and cracking of joints thirsty; unable to walk; **very weak**; left-sided sciatica; joint pains along with GI problems (diarrhea); **chilly**.

< cold damp, undressing
< 2–3 AM, after sleep
< hot weather
< alcohol, beer
< suppressed catarrh

> heat, motion

Kali carb (3)

Weakness, exhaustion; sharp neuralgic pain as if back were broken; low cervicals to sacrum, may get out of bed (3 AM) and walk around due to the pain; mainly L5 region, especially during pregnancy, miscarriage; difficulty walking; lying too long aggravates; sensation of a gnawing pain; discomfort in coccyx; **small of back feels weak**; **back and legs give out**; stiffness and paralytic feeling; pain in nates, thighs and hip joints; **pain from hips to knees**; **soles of feet very sensitive**; back and legs feel heavy; **sharp stitching pains**; burning in spine (Guaco); backache during and after miscarriage; **cramping in thighs and calves < night, early mornings and with walking**; backache pain < during and after movement; if perspiration and weakness are present due to the pains, think of Kali carb; thirsty and thirstless; **chilly**.

< cold air, water, drafts
< 2–3 AM; winter

> warm weather
> sitting with elbows on knees

< before menses
< on painful or left side
< loss of fluids; labor
< after coition

> open air
> leaning forward
> movement

Lachesis (2)

Right-sided sciatica (only time it is right); burning, shooting pain down leg to foot; pain with movement, marked anxiety and nervousness; **sensitive to pressure**; sensitive nape of neck; spasm of back muscles; weak back and knees, stoops when walking; coccyx pain is sharp, **worse rising from sitting posture**; must sit perfectly still; sensation of threads stretched from back to arms, legs, eyes, etc., sciatic pain better lying down, but may awake with it; **pain in tibia**; thirsty; chilly.

< sleep, after; AM
< heat, of room, sun, etc.
< empty swallowing
< slight touch
< noise; alcohol
< cloudy weather
< retarded discharges
< closing eyes
< pressure of clothes

> open air
> discharges
> hard pressure
> cold drinks

Lycopodium (3)

Burning pain between scapula; pain goes from right to left; burning pain in occiput; wants to be fanned on back while in spasm; left-sided sciatica = sore; tight or weak neck; knee pains, cramps in calves; similar to Rhus-tox but with Lycopodium mental/emotional; **cannot lie on painful side**; **sciatica < right side**; low back pain > heat, < first motion (Rhus t); gas, distention, bloating; thirstless; chilly.

< pressure of clothes
< warmth; waking; wind
< eating
< 4–8 PM

> warm food and drinks
> cold applications
> motion; eructations
> urinating
> after midnight

Nux vomica (3)

Tearing, constricting pain; **sits up to turn over due to pain**; burning in spine; sitting is painful; sudden loss of power in legs, arms in AM; sitting is painful; backache in lumbar region; mentals of Nux-vom; thirsty; **chilly**.

< 3–4 AM; overwork	> lying down
< walking, sitting	> free discharges
< cold, open air	> naps; wrapping head
< uncovering; noise	> hot drinks; warm

Oxalic acid (1)

Deep midscapular pain, burning, back feels numb; pain shoots along groin and thigh; **pain in spots** (Kali bich), **< thinking of the pains**; numb, weak backache; back feels too weak to hold body; **lancinating pains** shooting down extremities; pains start in spine and go down extremities.

< thinking about pain	> after stool
< touch; mental exertion	> light touch
< shaving	
< left side	

Plumbum (2)

Cannot support head, C5, C6, C7 upper thoracics; sharp neuralgic pains worse night; awake with headache, cervical muscles feel weak; right- or left-sided pain; low back pain to legs to posterior leg to foot; L1, L2 pain to abdomen; lightning-like pains; paralysis of lower extremities; disk injury; antispasmodic; muscle and thigh **pains come in paroxysms**; loss of patellar reflex; back ache worse bending backward; **retractions and indurations**; paralytic weakness (Curare); associated with progressive **muscle weakness**, **atrophy**, **paralysis**, **gout**; thirsty; chilly.

< at night; open air	> hard pressure
< clear weather	> rubbing
< exertion; motion	
< company; touch	
< grasping smooth objects	

Rhus tox (3)

Left side often; burning, tearing pains (Lyc); from heavy lifting, straining; stiffness of back and neck; **restless, can't rest in any position**; outer scapular pain worse swallowing; coccyx aches into thighs; cramps in calves; etiology—getting wet, over lifting, strains; **stiffness in small of back**; < from over work; **thirsty**; **cold**;

< wet, cold air
< chill; sitting
< hot and sweaty; uncovering
< beginning motion; **rest**
< before storms, overexertion
< after midnight
< during sleep; lying on right side

> continued motion
> heat; warm bath
> rubbing; change of position
> holding abdomen
stretching out limbs
> lying on a hard surface

Ruta (2)

Pain nape of neck, back, loins; legs give out when rising from chair (Con, Phos); lumbago worse in AM before rising; weakness of hips and thighs; hamstrings feel shortened (Graph); **thigh pain when stretching limbs**; **tendons sore**; thighs feel broken; pains deep in bones; cracking joints worse walking in open air; **any injury to tendons**; very restless; consider using in homeopathic tincture form.

< overexertion
< cold air; wind, damp
< lying; sitting
< pressure on an edge
< before arising in AM

> lying on back
> warmth
> motion
> pressure

Tellurium

Pain in sacrum which extends to right thigh and is < pressing at stool; aching in small of back; bruised pain in hip joints; sense of weight in back and sacrum; spine is sensitive and patient fears touch (Chin s, Phos); dull pain in vertebrae; pain runs from 7th cervical to 5th thoracic vertebrae; weak feeling in back; < coughing, sneezing and laughing; aching all over, mostly in limbs which is < on the right side with walking.

< touch
< coughing, laughing
< at rest
< lying on painful side

Viscum album

Chronic sciatica with much pain, along entire spine (neck to legs); **tearing**, shooting, throbbing pain; more left-sided; **glow rises from feet to head**; general tremors; severe sacral pain to pelvis **worse in bed** (Sulph); can't sleep with pain; itching all over; pains alternate between knee and ankle with shoulder and elbow.

< winter; cold
< stormy weather
< left side
< movement

Consider:

Arnica (3)

Sore, **bruised**, bed full of lumps; doesn't want to be touched; > lying.

Bryonia (3)

Painful stiffness of neck; cold; sacral pains with rigidity, can't walk upright; **> at rest**; shooting pain under left scapula > pressure; **< motion**; < during menses; > lying on painful side; < stooping.

Calcarea carb (3)

Rigid neck (L); dislocation-like pains; **from lifting**; hard to rise from sitting, shooting pains in shoulder blades; cold; exertion.

Causticum (2)

Back pain during menses; torticollis; violent lumbar pain; **< cold and damp**, pain above hips; < night, < lying; lameness of small back from a cold; > movement; painful stitching in back and sacrum, especially when rising from a chair; pain goes from sacrum to left hip which is tensive, as if the muscles are too short.

Cobalt (1)

Sciatica with nightly seminal emissions; < sitting; > walking or lying.

Coffea

Use with protrusion of the lumbar disk when patient is in severe pain, 10M dose as needed for pain.

Dulcamara (1)

Worse cold and damp, violent lumbar pain, pain above hips; < night, < lying; lameness of small back from a cold; > movement; pain as if sore or aching, mainly muscular after being drenched by rain.

Guaco

Irritation of the spine, with paralysis of lower extremities; pain along the spine; burning pains in the shoulders, extending to the forearms; hip pains with heaviness in the legs; consider for upper back, shoulder, arm and forearm pains; pains are < bending.

Guaiacum

Rheumatic pains, **especially of the head, neck and upper back**; **stiffness of neck and shoulders**; sciatica and lumbago; **sensation of heat in affected joints**; < motion, heat, cold weather, > pressure.

Natrum mur (3)

Sore neck, stiff, rigid, pain and paralysis in sacrum, especially in AM; shooting pain and pulsation in sacrum; weakness > lying, < eating; pain tears across loins and hips; **pain > lying on a hard surface**.

Natrum sulph (3)

Closed person, moody; > movement, > open air; < cold and damp; **headaches from head trauma**; stitches nape of neck at night; sore spine; tingling in calves; feet.

Phosphorus (3)

Burning in sacrum, between shoulder blades and in limbs; < storm or weather changes.

Silicea (3)

Weakness of muscles, paravertebral pain in low back; < cold drafts.

Staphysagria (2)

Feels as if back is broken, weak legs, compressive pains of low back; sciatica alternates with croupy cough; < rising from chair; psoas abscess.

Sulphur (3)

Sharp, along entire spine, burning pain; < cold, < standing; > stooping; > lying down; left side; cannot stand erect.

Thuja (1)

Painful drawing in sacrum and loins while sitting; can't stand erect on rising; left neck, SI pain extending to groin.

Symptoms in Kent's Repertory	**Page**
Back, Injuries of the spine	892
Back, Opisthotonus	893
Back, Pain, bending backwards agg./amel.	895
Back, Pain, coughing	895
Back, Pain, lifting	896
Back, Pain, lying/on back/amel.	897
Back, Pain, motion, on beginning to move	897
Back, Pain, sitting, while	897
Back, Pain, standing	898
Back, Pain, walking agg./amel.	899
Back, Pain, lumbar region	905
Back, Pain, lumbar region, motion	906
Back, Pain, lumbar region, rising from seat	907
Back, Pain, lumbar region, sacral	909
Back, Stiffness, sitting after	946
Back, Weakness, lumbar region	950

BRONCHITIS

Bronchitis is an acute inflammatory condition of the upper respiratory tract and is quite often preceded by a cold or flu. When the **cold** or **influenza** has evolved into bronchitis, it is often due to the improper treatment of giving anti-inflammatory agents and cough suppressants. Bronchitis by itself without a previous upper respiratory infection is rare.

The person may complain of low energy, chills, a low-grade fever, increased mucus discharge from the nose and throat, sore throat and chest and back pain or soreness. The cough may become more productive as the condition gets worse, and shortness of breath and wheezing may also occur.

The condition is usually self-limiting but without proper treatment may become chronic and appear similar to **emphysema**. Any change in the person's condition resulting in a greater difficulty with breathing should be referred to a physician as **pneumonia** can follow.

Early treatment with homeopathic medicines will help to quickly resolve this condition, but it is not unusual to see patients with a chronic cough following a bout of bronchitis. Nutritional support should be considered in these cases to help with regeneration of the bronchial mucosa.

Ammonium carb (1)

Elderly, chronic goes to acute; **cough with no expectoration**; incessant cough worse at night; cough occurs 3–4 AM; dyspnea; palpitations; burning of chest; **much oppression in breathing**; chronic emphysema; slow, labored, stertorous breathing; bubbling sound; pulmonary edema; sputum slimy with specks of blood; hoarseness; sense of heaviness in chest; chilly.

< evenings, lying	> lying on painful side,
< cold, wet weather	> dry weather

< wet applications
< 2–4 AM
< menses
< any effort
< entering warm room
< ascending steps

Antimonium tart (3)

Cyanotic, prostrated, rales throughout chest, wheezing respiration; must sit up to breathe; mucus in throat; violent tickle in trachea, cough loose-sounding; whole chest involved; gets chilly; flaring of nasal ala; weakness; cold; sweats; thickly coated white tongue; **great rattling of mucus but very little expectorated**; burning sensation in chest; **coughing and gasping at the same time**; **edema and impending paralysis of lungs**; emphysema of aged; hoarseness; rapid, short breaths; rapid pulse (Carbo veg); **thirstless.**

< evenings	> sitting up
< lying down at night	> eructations, expectoration
< warmth, cough and SOB	> lying on right side
< cold damp weather	(Badiaga opp.)
< milk, sour things	

Arsenicum alb (3)

Burning in chest; elderly; feeble; chilly; feeling of suffocation when lying down; fear of lying down; **of death**; exhausted; restless; **anxious**; dry violent cough; difficulty breathing afterward; thirst for sips of hot or cold; feeling of smoke in lungs (Brom); asthma worse at midnight; expectoration scanty; **frothy**; **darting pain through upper third of right lung**; wheezing respiration; hemoptysis with pain between shoulder blades; **thirsty for sips**; **chilly**.

< night	> heat
< wet weather	> head elevated
< cold; cold drinks; food	> warm drinks
< seashore	
< right side	

Belladonna (2)

Lethargic, stupor, delirium, perspires on covered parts; fever 103 or greater; bright red face with no perspiration; pupils dilated; **throat constricted**; **short**, **quick respiration**; **dry cough**; tickle in trachea; infant cries with cough; **no thirst**, **anxiety**, **fear**; hoarse, husky voice; small amount of sputum; **short cough**; Cheyne-Stokes respirations (Cocain, Op); painless hoarseness; barking cough with pain in stomach before attack; **larynx very painful**; **high piping voice**; **moans at every breath** (often follows Aconite, Ferrum phos); thirsty and thirstless.

< lying down	> semi-erect
< night, touch, jarring	
< drafts	
< after noon	

Bryonia (3)

Dryness; (later than Bell) beginning of effusion; dry mouth, parched lips; **thirst for cold**; dry hard cough may cause splitting headache; **grabs chest and sides with cough**; stitching pain with breathing; cough as if chest will fly apart (Phos); cough from tickle deep in sternum; has to sit up to cough; cough aggravated by eating, drinking, **entering a warm room** (Nat c); violent cough causes gagging; feverish; doesn't want to move; oppression in chest (Phos); little sputum; pleuritic pains; frequent desire to take long breaths, must expand lungs; difficult, quick respirations; touch mucus loosened by much coughing; soreness of larynx, trachea; **thirsty**.

< motion, **touch**	**> open windows**
< warmth, hot weather	**> lying on painful side**
< morning; eating	**> pressure**
< exertion	**> rest**; **cold**

Drosera (3)

Compression of chest; burning; stitches of pain; cough, with bright red sputum of clotted blood; **must press chest with hand for relief**; spasmodic, dry, irritative cough; **paroxysms follow one anoth-**

er very rapidly-whooping cough; can barely breathe-chokes; cough **deep and hoarse**; yellow expectoration **with bleeding from nose**, mouth; **retches due to cough**; sensation of crumbs or feather in throat; mucus in throat causes cough; coughs rapidly which may end in convulsions; patient breaks out in a cold sweat from coughing, is prostrated from cough; cough less during day but gets worse at night; must exert to speak; **asthma when talking**; bruised sensation in larynx with inspiration; voice is low and hoarse; restless, anxious, suspicious, fears being alone, ghosts; dread of nightmares; thirsty.

< after midnight	> drinking
< lying down	> singing, laughing
< getting warm in bed	
< cold food, drink	> motion

Hepar sulph (3)

Loose rattling cough, **chokes**; later stages of bronchitis; wheezing; little expectoration; but much mucus; difficult to get to come up; causes nausea and vomiting; **set off by dry**, **cold exposure**; has to bend backwards to keep breathing; **cough whenever any part of body gets cold or uncovered**; from eating cold food; hoarseness with loss of voice; cough when walking; anxious wheezing; heart palpitations; **very sensitive**; thirsty; **chilly**.

< cold, dry winds, drafts	> damp weather
< touch	> wrapping head
< lying on painful side	> warmth
	> after eating
	> hot drinks

Ipecac (3)

First stages of bronchitis-rapid effusion; onset from warm moist air; **increased secretions in throat**, **can't get it out**; rattling cough; rales over entire chest (louder than Ant-t); chest full of phlegm; wheezing; face is blue; violent dyspnea (less than Ant-t); tickling from larynx to bottom of bronchi; violent coughing spasms causes pale face; **retching and vomiting**; must sit up to breathe; **gags and nearly suffocates from mucus**; tough, thick mucus; yearly attacks;

constriction of chest; **cough incessant and violent with every breath**; bleeding from **lungs with nausea**; hemoptysis from slightest exertion (Millef); aphonia; persistent nausea; bright red hemorrhage which clots quickly; thirstless; chilly.

< lying down
< periodically
< moist warm wind; dry cold
< warm room
< evening, early night
< movement

> open air

Natrum sulph (3)

Dyspnea from damp weather; **holds chest when coughing** (Bry); rattling in chest, especially 4–5 AM, cough with thick, ropy, greenish expectoration; **feels every change from dry to wet**; constant desire to take deep long breath; pain through **lower left chest**; fresh cold brings on asthma attack; **empty**, **all-gone feeling in the chest**.

< music
< lying on left side
< dampness
< rainy and damp weather

> dry weather
> pressure, changing position

Phosphorus (3)

Subacute, lingering conditions; head cold that goes to lungs; constricted larynx with pain, can't talk; may have painless hoarseness; talking aggravates cough; cough from behind sternum; **cough so painful that they try to suppress it**; **oppression in chest**; cough is easier if sitting; bloody sputum-tastes salty or sweet; soreness, rawness of chest; constant desire to clear throat; **chilly**; **thirsty**; burning pains; sharp stitches in chest; **respiration rapid**, **oppressed**; **much heat in chest**; whole body trembles with cough; pneumonia; **thirst for cold**; **chilly**.

< talking, touch
< evenings to midnight
< after meals
< lying on left side
< weather changes

> in dark
> lying on right side
> cold food; cold
> open air
> washing with cold water

< ascending stairs
< warm food

Pulsatilla (3)

Cough with thick, bland, purulent yellow/green discharge; dry tickling cough; trachea irritated; foul odor in mouth (Merc); **must sit up in bed to get relief**; **loose cough in AM dry cough in PM**; **pressure upon chest and is sore**; short of breath; anxiety; palpitations when lying on left side (Phos); feels smothered with lying down; **thirstless**; **dry mouth**; **peevish**; **chilly**; sensitive; hoarseness comes and goes; **thirstless.**

< warm room, heat
< fats, rich foods
< evenings
< lying on left or painful side
< hanging feet down

> open air
> consolation
> motion
> cold applications, food, drink

Rumex (2)

Cough from inhaling very cold air; sense of lump in throat; no relief from hawking or swallowing; **rawness under clavicle**; cough from tickle in throat to bronchi; dry, hoarse, barking spasmodic cough; **cough with pain behind mid-sternum**; puts covers over head to stop cough; can't lie on left side; stitching pain in left lung; **copious mucus** from nose and trachea; cough **prevents sleep**; cough **aggravated by pressure**; **talking**; sputum is watery, thin, frothy to string and touch; chilly.

< evenings, 11 PM
< inhaling cold air
< lying on left side
< uncovering
< 5 AM (Nat sulph)

> covering mouth, wrapping up

Sanguinaria (3)

Lingering disease; dryness of airways; circumscribed redness on cheeks with cough; tickle in throat, sternal pain with cough (Bry, Phos, Rumex); sputum difficult, offensive, rust color; constricted chest; sighs constantly; burning pain in chest; **cough of gas-**

tric origin, better with eructations; burning soreness of right chest through right shoulder; **severe dyspnea**; must sit up to breathe; cough from exposure to cold; **sudden stopping of catarrh of respiratory tract followed by diarrhea**; aphonia; pneumonia better lying on back.

< sweets	> acids, sleep
< right side	> darkness
< motion, touch; lying down at night	

Spongia (3)

Dry bronchitis; wheezing; **anxiety**; difficulty in breathing; abnormal breath sounds which are dry and rattling, with a raw and scraped throat; hard dry cough; dyspnea; no sputum; **hoarseness**; **larynx dry**, **constricted and burns**; **barking**, **croupy cough**; **croup worse during inspiration**; short, panting, difficult respirations; plug-in-throat sensation; **cough abates after eating or drinking**; cough from deep in chest; **exhaustion**; **heaviness of body after slight exertion**; fear; great hunger; thirst; constant desire to clear throat.

< lying down, warm room	**> leaning forward**
< midnight to 4 AM	**> hot water**, **eating**
< ascending	> descending
< wind	> lying with head low

Stannum (3)

Chest feels raw, sore, hollow; mucus expelled by forcible cough; violent, dry cough evening until midnight; cough from **laughing**, talking, singing; cough worse lying on right side; **copious green**, **sweetish sputum**; chest feels weak; can hardly talk; respiration is short, oppressive; stitching pain on left side with breathing, lying on left side; **extreme weakness**; **pains increase gradually then slowly subside**; chilly.

< using voice	> coughing or expectorating
< lying on left side	> hard pressure
< warm drinks	> rapid motion
< after motion	
< ascending steps	
< 10 AM; cold	

Consider:

Aconite (2)

Onset from cold dry winds; anxious, fretful, restless; fever preceded by chills; hot dry skin; short, dry cough; aggravated by everything; watery and blood-streaked sputum; **hoarse dry croupy cough**; **oppressed breathing**; sensitive to inspired air; tingling in chest after cough; worse night, after midnight, lying on affected side; > open air; **thirsty**.

Balsam of Peru

Old folks; chronic bronchitis; loud rales over entire chest; **profuse thick**, **creamy yellow sputum** , cottage cheese-like; **night sweats with debility**; loose cough.

Carbo veg (2)

If Ant-t doesn't work; very cyanotic; opens windows and **wants to be fanned**; acute stages or chronic flare-ups; rattling in chest; shortness of breath; **burning in chest behind sternum**; spasmodic cough-sore chest; cough with itching in larynx; < evenings, warm damp weather, cold, fats, milk; > leaning forward; profuse yellow, fetid, sticky sputum, difficult to dislodge; thirsty; chilly.

Conium

Dry cough, < evening, night; **caused by a dry spot in larynx**, with **itching** in chest and throat **when lying down**, talking; **little sputum production which must be swallowed**.

Dulcamara (2)

From sudden changes in temperatures: hoarse, spasmodic cough; summer colds; cough caused by tickle in throat with much loose, easy expectoration, **cough after physical exertion**; may cough a long time to expel phlegm; bronchitis in children, < night, cold, damp rainy weather; > moving about, warmth; dry cough evolves into over producing much mucus; thirsty; **chilly**.

Ferrum phos (3)

Coughs then loses urine (Caust, Puls); **first stage of all inflammatory conditions**; congestion, hemoptysis; hard dry cough with sore chest; cough > at night; > cold applications, < night, 4–6 AM, motion; thirsty.

Mercurius (2)

Much catarrh; soreness and scraped sensation from back of throat to bronchi; tickle; dryness in chest causes cough; fluent watery or yellow purulent sputum; thirst for cold; dry mouth; indented tongue; yellow; chills alternate with fever; offensive breath; body odor; trembling tongue, protrusion; **cannot lie on right side**; cough < tobacco smoke; < night and warmth of bed; > moderate temperatures; thirst; chilly.

Senega—See under asthma.

Symptoms in Kent's Repertory	**Page**
Chest, Inflammation, bronchial tubes	835
Chest, Inflammation, lungs (pneumonia)	835
Chest, Inflammation, infants	836
Chest, Inflammation, pleura pneumonia	836
Chest, Edema, pulmonary	838
Chest, Oppression, when coughing	839
Chest Pain, inflammation of lungs, after	843
Chest Pain, inspiration during	843
Chest Pain, pressure amel.	843
Chest Pain, respirations deep	844
Chest Pain, sides, lungs	848
Expectoration, Bloody	813
Expectoration, Copious	814
Expectoration, Difficult	815

See rubrics under **Croup** for type of cough.

BURNS

Burns and **scalding** of the skin may result from a variety of sources such as the sun, heating units, hot liquids, electrical sources, chemical agents or radiation. The degree of burn will be dependent upon the duration and intensity of exposure.

A **first-degree burn** damages the outer layer of skin, resulting in redness and sensations of heat and pain. This is commonly seen with a sunburn. A **second-degree burn** results in damage that lies below the upper layer of skin extending into the dermis. Along with redness and pain, vesicles or blisters will form. **Third-degree burns** destroy both the upper and lower layers of skin along with nerve endings, resulting in pain initially followed by numbness. These are the **most severe type of burns** that result in loss of fluids, which can lead to shock and possibly death.

Second- and third-degree burns require medical supervision, as continued loss of fluid through the burn site can result in electrolyte imbalance and a decreased plasma volume. This leads to dehydration and shock. Bacterial infection also occurs whenever there is disruption of the skin and dead tissue present.

Arsenicum alb (3)

Skin which appears as if it has been **seared**, with less of the epithelial surface, in small scales or large flakes; chronic **burning** ulcerations; skin is red, swollen and very sensitive to touch; dark metallic like discoloration, black and blue spots; skin which is **dry**, **rough**, **scaly**; **prostration** which may seem out of proportion to severity of condition; **restlessness**, especially with the pains; **chilly**; bleeding from inflamed areas; burning pains with ichorous, offensive discharge; **thirsty**.

< cold
< midnight, after 3 AM

> warmth

Cantharis (3)

Burns and **scalds** with a feeling of painful rawness which is > with cold applications, may be followed by much inflammation; biting raw pains or **cutting, burning or smarting pains**; eruptions which burn with being touched; burning sensation of the skin before blister formation; small vesicles which coalesce to form larger blisters; weakness and faintness with a feeble pulse; shuddering with external coldness; delirium; suddenness of onset of symptoms (Bell) with a rapid progression; for burns, scalds, sunburn; **extensive burns causing renal involvement**.

< coffee	> warmth
< movement; touch	> rest

Carbolic acid (1)

Sensation of heat, tingling and numbness of the skin; may also be painful, with eventual progression to a dry gangrene; violet discoloration of the skin; inflammation of the skin with sloughing; patient may have vomiting and diarrhea; offensive discharges; **rapid prostration with coldness of the skin resulting in shock and collapse**; vesicles which itch and are relieved by rubbing, which is followed by burning; will tend to ulcerate; thirsty.

< strong odors	> rubbing (itching)
< cold air	

Carbo veg (2)

Ecchymosis of the skin, **coldness**, **blueness**, rawness, ulcerations which are foul, burning and bleed easily, which have a tendency to heal then form again; burning pains which are felt in inflamed parts as well as in veins and capillaries of the skin; **sluggishness of circulation** causing oozing of dark colored blood which will not clot; fine, moist rash with burning in spots; pooling of blood in areas laid upon with numbness and ulcer formation; patient may chill and require cold drinks (Ign) but ceases to be thirsty with the return of the fever; exhausting sweats; ***patient wishes to be fanned even though chilly;*** will feel burning internally but cold externally; good medicine for shock, sepsis.

< evenings	**> being fanned**
< depletions, of fluids	**> cool air**

Causticum (2)

Rawness and soreness, **fissures** and **cracks** in the skin, especially at the corners of the mouth, nose and eyes (Nit ac); thick, dry skin with scabs and crusts, especially on back of the head; **itching** eruptions with soreness and rawness; perspiration is sour smelling which can occur from becoming heated or with walking; **effects of deep burns**; breakdown of old injuries, scars, especially old burns.

< extremes of temperature (Merc)	**> damp**, **wet weather**
< dry, cold, **wind**	

Kreosotum (2)

Eruption of large pustule-like rash or wheals, vesicular eruption with violent itching; scratching does not make the itch better but causes a burning sensation; < 5 to 7 PM or night; ecchymosis (Carbo veg), wounds bleed easily (Crot, Lach, Phos).

< rest; touch	> warmth
< cold	> open air

Urtica urens—see **Stings of Insects**

Symptoms in Kent's Repertory	**Page**
Skin, Erysipelas, gangrenous	1323
Skin, Gangrene, from burns	1325
Generalities, Blackness, of external parts	1346
Generalities, Burns	1346
Generalities, Loss of fluids	1371
Generalities, Septicemia	1399

CANKER SORES—GLOSSITIS—TRENCHMOUTH

Commonly referred to as **canker sores**, these painful ulcerations of the oral mucosa may occur singly or in groups. The cause is not known but thought to be due to stress or allergies to foods. Deficiencies of iron, vitamin B_{12} or folic acid must be considered, especially if there is a poor response to therapy.

Ulcerations begin as a vesicle but quickly become a shallow, ovoid erosion with a slightly raised border surrounded by a narrow, dark red zone. The ulceration usually is covered over by a whitish to yellow membrane within 5 to 7 days. With severe attacks there may be numerous ulcerations accompanied by fever, low energy and enlarged lymph nodes. Attacks may be recurrent in nature, occurring several times per year.

Generally **aphthous ulcers** are not considered a medical emergency but can become severe enough that it is difficult for the person to eat or drink. If lesions are preceded by a high fever, then other conditions such as **erythema multiforme** need to be considered.

Arsenicum alb (3)

Crohn's disease with ulcers in mouth; **ulcers burn like fire**; borders of tongue affected; offensive odor; grey/white ulcers at first going to purple/blue to black (gangrene of mouth); **very restless**; gums bleed easily; ulcers dry with burning heat; tongue is dry, clean, red; metallic taste; **drinks in sips**, **warm water**; **desires cold drinks but aggravate oral lesions**; **anguish**; **fear of death**, **sudden great weakness**, **chilly**.

< cold drinks, foods, air
< after midnight, 2 AM
< exertion, tobacco
< lying
< suppressed eruptions

> warm drinks, applications
> motion
> elevating head, sitting erect
> company, sweating

Baptisia (3)

Similar to Lachesis; **putrid-smelling** (more than Merc); oral mucosa is dark, purplish, red color; great salivation; **all right drinking water but can't eat food** (painful); cracked tongue, especially middle; swollen glands; taste is flat, bitter; **tongue feels burned**; thick speech; insensible to pain; feels dull and confused; viscid salivation, ragged ulcerations; thirsty.

< humid heat; fog
< pressure
< on awaking
< in a room

Borax (3)

Increased sensitivity, especially to cutting flavors (acids); mouth hot and dry, red mucus, will bleed if touched; may get blisters on tongue (Nat mur), occur mainly on inside of cheek and tongue; mouth feels dry but saliva present; lst remedy for thrush (white plaque with red base), **very sensitive to pain and noise**. **Dread of downward motion**; anxiety on face; baby can't nurse, will vomit with eating or drinking; child is pale, pasty face with green-yellow diarrhea, white fungus-like growth; things taste bitter (Bry, Cupr, Puls); thirsty.

< salt, spicy food	> 11 PM
< downward motion	
< sudden noises	
< cold, wet ; least uncovering	
< nursing ; fruit	

Kali chl (3)

Mucus membranes red with grey-based ulcers; sometimes both sides of tongue near front; tongue with grey fur; submandibular swelling (Merc); cold with white mucus; **fetid mouth**, grayish-white exudates; noma = ulcerative stomatitis; profuse secretion of acid saliva; **gangrenous ulcers**.

< cold
< mercury

Lachesis (2)

Swollen gums, spongy, bleed; tongue is swollen, trembling, burns, red, dry with a cracked tip; **ulcers**, **denuded spots** (lying bare); burning and rawness; nauseous taste; **left-sided complaints**; thick speech; tongue catches on teeth; thirsty; chilly.

< sleep, heat	> open air
< swallowing	> discharges
< slight touch, pressure	> hard pressure, cold drinks

Mercurius cor (3)

Similar to Merc; **develops very quickly**, fast tissue destruction, burning of whole mouth; ulcers on palate; increased tenesmus with stool; gums purple, swollen and spongy; swollen inflamed tongue, salivation, pyorrhea; **gums bleed easily**, bleeding mucosal lesions (has more of a border, deeper than Merc viv); **astringent taste**, **dysphagia**, insatiable thirst.

< after stool; urinating
< swallowing
< night, cold, autumn
< hot days, cool nights
< acids

Mercurius sol. or Mercurius viv (3)

Foul taste of metallic, bitter, putrid, salty, sour; **intense salivation**; swollen glands; foul odor; ulcer, usually no border, very superficial; thirst for cold drinks; burning of ulcers, especially at night; constant desire to swallow; sensitive to temperature changes; profuse perspiration which doesn't help fever, throws covers off; **increased thirst with a moist mouth**; **spongy gums**, **tongue**; bleeding gums; **indented tongue**.

< night	
< sweating; heated	
< lying on right side	
< wet feet	
< weather changes	
< drafts to head	> moderate temperature

Muriatic acid (3)

Tongue is pale, swollen, dry, leather-like appearance; deep ulcers on tongue ; gums and glands swollen; fetid breath; **sordes on teeth** (fetid, brown crusts), hard lumps in tongue; **restless**, (increased nervousness) leading to becoming weak (Ars); **burning ulcers**; bluish ulcers, tongue; lips sore and cracked, scabs.

< touch; sitting	> motion, warmth
< wet weather, bathing; cold drinks	
< walking	> lying on left side
< alcohol, morning	

Natrum mur (2)

Dry mouth, lips cracked in middle; **excoriating vesicles around mouth**; intense dryness of ulcers; **geographic tongue** (Ars, Rhus t, Tarax); **after sharp foods edges of tongue get hard**; feeling of hair on tongue; **numbness and tingling of tongue**, lips; **herpes of lips**; blunted taste; mild thirst or in large quantities; **craves salt**, chilly.

< 9–11 AM, sun, heat	> open air, cold bathing
< exertion, emotions	> sweating, rest
< sympathy	> deep breathing
	> early AM

Nitric acid (2)

Gums look pale, swollen; sharp needle-like pains, Merc tongue, swollen, indented; profuse salivation which is acrid and excoriates the lips (more than Merc); sensitive to cold, bloody acrid discharges; irritable, especially in AM; moist, fissured or mapped tongue; flabby sore gums; putrid breath; painful pimples on side of tongue ; **fissures at corners of mouth or other mucocutaneous borders**; irritable, angry, hateful, profane, **anxiety for health**; **chilly**.

< slight touch, jarring	> gliding motions, riding
< noise, motion	> mild weather
< cold, after eating	> steady pressure
< dampness, night	
< weather changes	
< heat of bed, exertion	

Nux vomica (3)

Small aphthous ulcers with bloody saliva; posterior tongue covered with fur; gums swollen, white and bleeding; taste is bitter, sour; fits the generals of Nux-vom; thirsty, **chilly**.

< early AM	> free discharges
< cold, open air, drafts	> heat
< uncovering	> resting
< coffee, stimulants	> wrapping head
< overeating	
< mental overexertion	
< noise, odors, touch	
< pressure of clothes	

Sulphuric acid (3)

Wasting disease, alcohol abuse; **ulcers bleed with touch**—dark blood; greenish/black (Ledum), dark bloody salivation, sour vomiting; **tremor**, disproportionate weakness; hemorrhage; sourness; very painful; black and blue spots—petechiae; fretful, impatient, consider if Borax doesn't work; chilly.

< open air, cold drinks	> hot drinks
< odor of coffee	> heads near head
< evenings	> moderate temperatures
< excessive hot or cold	> motion, lying on affected side

Sulphur (3)

Similar to Borax, dryness, burning, heat, **red lips**, thirst for cold drinks; **bitter taste in AM**; swollen gums; throbbing pain; tongue white with red tip and borders; sore mouth from nursing; chilly.

< suppressions, bathing	> open air, motion
< heated, speaking	> warm applications
< atmospheric changes	> sweating, dry heat
< 11 AM, full moon	
< rest; **warmth of bed**; alcohol	

Consider:

Aethusa (2)

Aphthae from milk intolerance in infants; burning and pustules in throat with difficulty swallowing.

Cantharis (1)

Burning of mouth, throat and pharynx; vesicles cover tongue, mouth; **difficulty swallowing liquids**; very thick mucus.

TONGUE INFLAMMATION

Antimonium crud

Thrush remedy, tongue coated thick white; gums detached easily from teeth, bleed easily; **canker sores**; no thirst.

Apis (3)

Fiery red tongue, swollen, sore, raw, with vesicles; tongue feels scalded, red hot, trembling; mouth and tongue **red, shining and puffy**; < heat, > cold.

Crotalis c (3)

Scarlet tongue; paralysis of tongue; burning and pricking at tip; itching; saliva is thick, viscid, dark; white mucus discharge from mouth; salty taste; difficult speech; pains < night, < cold.

Crotalis h (3)

Tongue is very red, smooth, polished; feels swollen (Apis); protruded tongue which goes to the right; fetid breath; sore mouth; bloody or frothy salivation; < AM on awaking (Lach); tight or constricted feeling; < open air; difficulty swallowing solids (opp Lach), more right-sided than Lachesis.

GUM INFLAMMATION

Kreosotum (3)

Spongy, bleeding gums, with rapid tooth decay; teeth feel raised, with dull, throbbing pains; teeth are dark, crumbling; lips are red, bleed; putrid odor of mouth (Ant c, Staph); < cold, open air:

> warmth; ulcerations on tongue and buccal mucosa; burning sensation at angles of the mouth.

Petroleum (3)

Foul breath, sometimes smells like garlic; ulcers on inner surface of cheeks, painful, < closing mouth; white-coated tongue (Ant c); painful soreness with chewing.

Phosphorus (3)

Swollen and easily bleeding gums; tongue **dry**, **smooth**, **red** or white and not thickly coated; **thirst for cold water**.

Symptoms in Kent's Repertory	**Page**
Mouth Aphthae	397
Mouth, Bleeding	397
Mouth, Dryness thirst, with	403
Mouth, Dryness, thirstless	403
Mouth, Inflammation, palate	406
Mouth, Odor	409
Mouth, Pain, see appropriate rubric	410
Mouth, Pustules	415
Mouth, Saliva offensive	416
Mouth, Stomacace	420
Mouth, Spongy, gums	420
Mouth, Ulcers	428
Mouth, Ulcers, gums	428

CARDIAC PAIN—CHEST PAIN

Remedies listed under this section were selected primarily for the treatment of **angina** or **heart attack**. Certainly other conditions such as pneumonia, bronchitis, hiatal hernia and gastric ulcer, to name a few, may cause similar symptoms. Chest pains should be considered medical emergencies until proven otherwise and must be evaluated immediately by a physician. In these conditions, time is of the essence as delayed treatment may make recovery more difficult.

Treatment with homeopathic medicines while in transit to an emergency facility has been credited with saving more than one life, but as with any serious life threatening illness, more than one prescription may be necessary.

Aconite (3)

Panic, **fear of death**; numbness and tingling radiating down left arm; **restless**; lancinating pains keep patient from moving; **tachycardia**; left shoulder pain; tingling in fingers; pulse is **full**, **hard**, **tense**, **bounding**, temporal and carotid arteries felt when sitting; **sudden**; **violent** onset; **very sensitive to noises**; **burning thirst**.

< movement, touch	> open air, repose
< lying on affected side	> warm sweat
< dry cold winds	
< chills, night	
< emotions	
< warm room	

Cactus grand (3)

Constriction; tight pressing-down pain; **contraction**; **congestion**; cardiac pain goes to left abdomen; catches breath with pain; left ventricular hypertrophy; edema and cyanosis of face; **endocarditis with mitral insufficiency**; **violent and rapid action**; **constriction as if from an iron band around heart/chest**; palpitations; angina pectoris; pain shoots down left arm; tobacco heart; vertigo; dyspnea; flatulence; pulse is feeble, irregular, quick; endocardial murmurs; low blood pressure; sensation of a weight on chest; red-faced; head congestion > pressure.

< lying on left side; occiput	> open air
< exertion, periodically	> pressure on vertex
< 10–11 AM or 11 PM	
< ascending stairs	

Cenchris (3)

Dyspnea, mental and physical restlessness; wants clothes loose (Lach, Nux v); desires small sips of water; heart feels distended and fills whole chest; feels as if it is falling down in abdomen; sharp stitches; fluttering under left scapula.

< pressure; lying down
< afternoon, night

Cereus b (3)

Convulsive pain in heart; pains in chest through heart and spleen; pain in left pectoral muscle and left lower rib cartilage; sensation of a great weight on heart and prickling pain; hypertrophy of heart; difficult respiration as from compression of chest.

Digitalis (2)

Spasmodic, incomplete contractions; irregular pulse, beat, vertigo; spasmodic cough; can't lie down due to anguish from dyspnea; **sensation as if heart would cease if they moved** (Gels opp), **weakness**, **dilation of the heart**; gone feeling in chest; **irregular**; **slow beats** (Apo, Can, Kalm), **quickened by least movement**; cardiac failure after fever; pericarditis; copious serous secretion; **patient must walk about**; skin is cold, clammy, doughy appearance; nausea; **cannot bear to talk due to dyspnea**; desire to take deep breath; **thirsty**; chilly.

< rising up, exertion	> rest, cool air
< lying on left side; heat	> lying flat on back
< smell of food; cold drinks	> empty stomach
< after meals; music	> lying still

Glonoine (2)

Increased throbbing of heart, rapid pulse with much force, throbbing neck vessels; **alternating congestion heart and head**; laborious action of heart; fluttering; palpitation with dyspnea; exertion brings on rush of blood to heart and fainting spells; patient is confused, bewildered; sun stroke; **waves of terrible bursting, pounding headache**; cardiac pains radiate to arms; full tense pulse; violent palpitations < stooping; patient must lie with head held high.

< leaning backward
< lying on left
< heat on head, overheating
< motion; hair cuts
< wine, fruits
< stooping
< 6 AM to noon

> open air; cold
> lying on right
> elevating head
> cold applications, bathing

Kalmia latifolia (3)

Weak, slow pulse (Apoc, Can, Dig); feeble, irregular heart beat; fluttering of heart; **palpitation worse leaning forward**; gouty and rheumatic heat; tachycardia with pain (Thyr), tobacco heart; **sharp pains take away breath**; shooting pain through chest above heart into shoulder blades; frequent pulse; tumultuous, rapid and visible heart action; pains change from place to place rapidly, come and go rapidly (Bell); pains may begin in limbs and go to heart; thirst; chilly.

< leaning forward
< looking down
< motion; open air
< heat of sun (pains)

> eating
> cloudy weather
> continued motion

Latrodectus mactans (2)

Consider as a first remedy to give for myocardial infarctions; constricting feeling; screams out from pain; violent precordial pain with numbness into extremities; **angina pectoris**; pain extends into and down left arm; pulse feeble and rapid; sinking at epigastrium; **restless, gasps for breath**; may have pain to both arms (Kalm); cold skin.

< least motion; exertion

Spigelia (3)

Sharp, stabbing pain, radiating up then down right or left arm, through heart; pain followed by numbness; tremulous sensation in chest; much dyspnea with a change in position; violent palpitations; aggravated by movement; foul odor of breath; pulse is weak, irregular; pericarditis with sticking pains; rheumatic carditis; craving for hot water which relieves; **dyspnea**, **must lie on right side which relieves**, **with head high**; chilly.

- < touch; motion
- < tobacco, coition
- < raising arms; periodically
- > lying on right side
- > inspiration

Spongia (2)

Sensation of heart swelling as if it will explode; **awakes from sleep after midnight with pain and suffocation**; stinging, pressing precordial pain; **surging of heart into chest as if it would be forced out upward**; hypertrophy of heart; valvular insufficiency; flushed, hot and frightened (Acon); angina pectoris, faintness, anxious, sweating; difficulty lying down but feels better in horizontal position.

- < dry, cold wind
- < exertion; awakened
- < raising arms
- < before 12 midnight; ascending
- > lying with head low
- > eating a little
- > descending

Tarentula h (2)

Extreme restlessness; fear of death; air hunger; **sensation as if heart turned and twisted around**; pain as if squeezed or compressed, also in aorta, under left clavicle and down into umbilicus; throbbing of heart, arteries; palpitations; **alternate chills and heat**; **restless, though movement aggravates**; lack of control, sudden mood changes, spine sensitive to touch; profuse sweating, **sensitive to music**; **thirsty**; chilly.

- < motion, noise, cold
- < periodically
- > rubbing, sweating
- > open air; music
- > in sun; bright colors

Veratrum alb (1)

Tumultuous, irregular contractions; red face on lying down which pales with sitting up; anxious palpitations; **profound prostration, sudden excessive evacuations**; tobacco heart from chewing, etc; pulse irregular, feeble, hands cold, clammy; **thirsty**.

< exertion, drinking	> hot drinks; covering
< cold drinks	> walking about
< during pain	> lying; warmth
< night	

Consider:

Coffea

Nervous palpitations with frequent urination; strong, quick heart beat from nervousness; rapid pulse.

Gelsemium

Feeling as if heart wold stop beating if he didn't move (Dig opp); slow pulse; nervous chill yet skin is warm; palpitations; pulse slow when quiet but rapid with motion; **weak slow pulse of old age**; **thirstless**.

Graphites (2)

Cold feeling around heat; sensation as if electric shock runs from heart to front of neck; < motion.

Kali bic (2)

Cold feeling around heart; pricking pain in cardiac region; tightness of chest; dilation, especially from kidney lesion; thirst; **chilly**.

Lachesis (3)

Sensation as if heart too large for chest; oppressive pain; expansion of heart as if in a full wind; palpitation with fainting spells; cyanosis; symptoms during climacteric; thirst; chilly.

Lilium tig (2)

Sensation as if heart in a vice (Cact); pulsations all over body; palpitations rapid; irregular pulse; sensation of load on chest; chest pains; cold feeling around heart; feels suffocated in a crowded, warm room; angina pectoris with pain in right arm or left arm; pains < stooping, < lying on right; < warmth; > cool, fresh air.

Lobelia (2)

Sensation as if heart would stand still; deep pain in and above heart; constriction or oppressive fullness of chest; weak pulse.

Phosphorus (2)

Diseases of right heart, venous stasis; tightness across chest with cough; systolic bellows murmur at base of lungs; violent palpitations with anxiety while lying on left side; rapid, soft, small pulse, dilated heart, especially right; feeling of warmth in heart; **thirst for cold**.

Phytolacca (1)

Shocks of pain shooting into right arm; feeling as if heart went to throat; weak heart action; < with expiration.

Rumex (1)

Feeling as if heart stopped; < with lying and has to sit up; red puffy face, especially around eyes; burning in heart; prostration; violent dry cough with tickle in throat; chilly.

Veratrum viride (2)

Pulse **slow, soft, weak**, irregular, intermittent; rapid pulse (Tabac, Dig), constant dull, burning pain in heart; valvular diseases; **pulses beat throughout body**, especially right thigh.

Symptoms in Kent's Repertory	**Page**
Chest, Angina pectoris	822
Chest, Anxiety, heart, region of	823
Chest, Constriction as from a band	826
Chest, Constriction heart	828
Chest, Fatty degeneration of heart	832
Chest, Fullness heart	833
Chest, Hypertrophy of heart	835

COLITIS—ABDOMINAL PAIN

See introduction under Abdominal Inflammation, above.

Aloe

Similar to Sulphur; stool gushes forth with great gurgling; great weakness; sputtering of flatus with mucus and stool; yellow clumps; 6 AM diarrhea; feel they want to pass gas but get stool; weakness around anus, can't hold stool back; **pain in rectum after stool**; **burning in anus and rectum**; constipation with pressure in lower abdomen; pain around navel < pressure; **abdomen feels heavy**, **hot**, **bloated**; **weak feeling as if diarrhea will come**; **sensation of plug between symphysis pubis and os coccygeus**; colic before and during stool; stool passes unnoticed; **sense of weakness in anus**; **venous congestion**; **heavy dragging**.

< heat; damp, summer	> cold, open air
< early AM; after dysentery	> cold applications
< stepping hard; evening	
< after eating and drinking	

Arsenicum alb

Intense tenesmus with severe burning; cutting, burning pain up rectum; stool excoriates and leaves anus red; **scanty dark blood in stool**; watery, involuntary; stinky, offensive, debilitating stools; **liver and spleen enlarged and painful**; ascites and anasarca; swollen, painful abdomen, dysentery; cholera stools; **restless**, **anxiety**, **fear of death**, fears, **anxiety about health**; mouth burning hot and dry; symptoms come on immediately after eating; **putrid**, **cadaveric odor**; **craves ice cold water which distresses**; **drinks little and often**; **thirsty**; cold externally; **chilly**,

< cold food and drink	> heat; head elevated
< after midnight, every 14 days	> warm drinks

< vegetables, drinking
< eruptions, bad meat
< tobacco; exertion
< lying on part
< wet weather; seashore

> motion
> company; sweating

Cantharis

Intense burning, scanty stools and urine; tenesmus in bladder and rectum with much urgency; burning, **intense thirst but are adverse to water**; stool mucus, blood, frothy; **shuddering** (Caps) **with burning of stool**; **aggravated by coffee**; **cutting**, **smarting pains**; **violent acute inflammation**; thirsty.

< urinating; touch
< cold drinks
< sound of water; night
< bright objects

> warmth; rest
> rubbing

Capsicum

Chronic dysenteries; chronic straining due to hemorrhoids; burning tenesmus in bladder and rectum; much gas; clutching, gripping pain; **much mucus and blood**; tenesmus and burning after stool; drinks cold water and gets chills all over body; **craves ice water**, **drawing pain in back after stool**; **thirst after stool with shivering**; **nose and face red but cold**; homesick; changeable, capricious; waterbrash; **thirsty**; **drinking causes shuddering**.

< slight drafts
< cold air, water
< uncovering, dampness
< bathing; empty swallowing
< urination; eating; drinking

> continued motion
> eating
> from heat

China

Whole abdomen distended like a drum; gas doesn't ameliorate passed either direction; much borborygmus; incarcerated gas; worse **fruit**, milk, beer; stools yellow, slimy to watery; can double up with pain; much thirst; profuse perspiration with diarrhea; **twisting pain about navel**; thirst aggravates diarrhea; white mucus like small pieces of popped corn, stool preceded by colic, **itching of anus**; **lienteric stool**; dark, foul, watery, **bloody stools**; **profuse sweating at night**, **exhausting discharges**; weak, oversensitive, nervous; **thirst and thirstless**; chilly; resembles Carbo veg but has stool often only at night with none during the day.

< loss of vital fluids	> hard pressure
< touch, noise, jarring	> loose clothing
< alternate days	
< cold, drafts, wind	
< open air, mental exertion	
< fruit, milk	
< looking fixedly at objects	
< sun, summer, night	

Colocynthis

Gas so severe it makes one **double over with pain**; digs elbows into stomach; pain increases in severity; acute or chronic conditions; **stools jelly-like**, ropy, stringy, like water, sensation as if stones being ground together and would burst; abdomen feels bruised, cramps in calves with colic; cutting pains especially after anger; pain in small spot just below navel; **dysenteric stool occurs every time patient eats or drinks**; stool has musty odor; distention; **sudden cramps**; pressure > at first then <; thirsty.

< emotions, vexation, anger	**> doubling over**
< lying on painless side	**> hard pressure**
< PM, in bed, drafts	> coffee, heat, rest
< taking cold; dentition	> gentle motion
	> after stool or flatus

Lycopodium

Pain on left side; severe cutting pains; hypogastrium; **starts on left and goes to right**; **with slightest food they bloat to painful tympanic abdomen**; sour eructations which temporarily relieve; severe colic which is cutting, clutching, gripping gas in stomach flexure on left side; borborygmus; aggravated by cold water and cold in general; constant sense of fermentation in abdomen; right side hernias; ineffectual urging for stool; **hard**, **difficult small incomplete**

stool; **full of gas**; **awakes angry**; incomplete eructations; colicky babies < evenings; thirstless, chilly.

< pressure of clothes
< warmth, awaking
< wind; indigestion; eating
< oysters; **4–8 PM**
< right side
< above to downward

> eructations
> motion
> warm drinks
> cold applications
> urinating

Mercurius cor

Intense tenesmus continues into bladder, worse at night; very little stool comes out, burns and cuts anus with passing, always bloody with mucus and pus; intense pain for hours; high fever with cold sweat; salivation, foul odor of mouth and stool; trembling of extremities; flushes of cold; bruised sensation, bloated and very painful to touch; tenesmus not > with stool; continuous urging for stool; **feels as if he is not done passing stool**; **dysphagia**; thirsty.

< after stool, urinating
< night, cold, autumn
< hot damp, cool nights
< acids
< swallowing

> resting

Mercurius sol

Similar to Mer cor but not as severe; get more stool with less straining; tenesmus over a longer period of time; watery, foul diarrhea; **goose flesh begins at feet and goes to head and back to feet**; excoriating stool; abscesses; associated with liver soreness and occasional diarrhea.

< night

Nux vomica

Intense clutching and **desire for stool but can't**, symptoms get worse; gripping pain in ascending colon; irregular colon peristalsis; diverticulitis; mucus passed; intense backache; needs to lie in hot water; **bruised soreness of abdomen**; flatulent distention; colic from uncovering; **weakness of abdominal ring region**; **stool feels as if part remains in rectum**; **absence of all desire is a contraindication**; **soreness < stepping or coughing**; **constant uneasiness in rectum**; covers up in bed; dysentery is aggravated by drugs; **irritable**, **angry**; **impatient**; **nervous**; thirst; **chilly**.

< early AM, open air	**> free discharges**
< cold, uncovering	> naps
< effects of high living	> wrapping head
< coffee; dry cold weather	> hot drinks; milk
< sedentary habits, mental exertion	> moist air
< disturbed sleep, noise	> strong pressure
< anger, odors, pressure of clothes	
< touch; light; spices	

Phosphorus

Irritation and infection of mucous membranes; intense burning pains, burning anus, fermentation, gurgling; whole abdomen distended and rumbling; watery stools, **fetid stools with flatus**, **great weakness after stool**, **painless debilitating diarrhea**; white hard stools; desire for stool lying on left side; involuntary stool, slender stool; rectal sensation of being open; sharp cutting abdominal pains; **weak**, **empty**, **gone sensation of abdominal cavity**; stool yellow, watery; **awakes at 5–6 AM** (Aloe); **craves cold drinks which are > but vomited when warm in stomach**; rubs abdomen to make it >; **thirsty for cold drinks**, **chilly**.

< lying on left side, painful side	
< odors	> sleep
< slightest emotions, touch	> cold food, water to face
< warm food and drink, salt	> rubbing (magnetized)
< sexual excesses	> sitting up; lying on right
< windy, cold, weather	
< weather changes, thunderstorms	
< AM & PM	

Pulsatilla

Much colic; distention, changeable stools; stool with yellow/green mucus; diarrhea alternates with constipation; bloody mucus

(Merc, Rheum); loud rumbling; pressure as if from a stone; diarrhea < night, after fruit (Ars, China); **two or three normal stools daily**; **averse to fats**, **water**; craves acids or disagreeable things; **emotional**, **weepy**, **shifting symptoms**; **timid**, **mild**, **thirstless**.

< warmth of room, clothes, air, bed	**> open air**, **cold**
< getting feet wet	**> erect posture**,uncovering
< suppressions, **evenings**, **rest**	> gentle motion, continued motion
< beginning motion, **lying**	> after a good cry
< rich foods, fats, eggs	
< before menses	
< lying on left or painless side	
< allowing feet to hang down	

Rhus tox

Tenesmus goes down leg; much watery, bloody stool; violent pain > lying on abdomen; swelling of inguinal glands; pain in ascending colon; colic causes him to walk doubled over; excessive distention after eating; rumbling of flatus on first rising but disappears with motion; red tip of tongue; **difficult to rest in any position** (Ars); stool smells cadaverous, like decomposing matter; frothy painless stools; **thirsty**; **chilly**.

< exposure to wet, **cold**, **washing**	> continued motion
< chill, draft; hot and sweaty	> heat
< uncovering; sleep	> rubbing
< beginning motion, **rest**	> holding abdomen
< after midnight, overexertion	> nose bleeds

Sulphur

Ineffectual urging; burning pains; excoriated **red anus**; stools yellow, mucus, gelatinous, acrid, bloody, slimy; abdomen is sensitive to pressure, feels raw and sore; colic after drinking; movement as if something is alive (Croc, Thuja); **morning diarrhea drives him out of bed**; won't pass stool due to pain; flushes of heat, needs windows open; abdomen > pressure; may have painless diarrhea; gray, frothy stools; similar to Aloe; **untidy**, **unkempt**, **sudden hunger < 11 AM**; **thirsty**; chilly.

< 5–6 AM
< suppressions; **bathing**
< milk
< heated; climacteric
< atmospheric changes
< speaking; 11 AM, full moon
< rest; standing
< alcohol; night

> open air; motion
> warm applications
> sweating; dry heat
> lying on right side
> drawing up affected limbs

See **Symptoms** under **Abdominal Inflammation**.

CONJUNCTIVITIS

Conjunctivitis may be caused by a virus, bacteria, allergy to environmental materials, or irritation from a foreign body. It is a common cause of eye disorders in children, and if viral in nature, can be highly contagious. Allergy to environmental materials includes smoke, chemicals (especially from swimming pools), pollens and dust. Bright lights from sun lamps or snow may also cause the condition. If irritation from a foreign body is suspected, the person needs to be examined by a physician to make sure that the cornea has not been damaged.

The person affected may complain of itching, stinging or foreign-body sensation in the eye. The eye itself will show redness and may have a mucoid or purulent discharge. The eyelids may stick together, especially in the morning upon awaking. There may be a large amount of tearing or blinking associated with the condition, which is the body's way of soothing the irritation to the eye. The person's vision is not usually affected, although it may become so with a chronic viral infection.

Aconite (3)

From foreign bodies; sudden onset; **dry**, **burning heat**; **much pain and restlessness**, **fearful**; after exposure to extreme heat or cold; one cheek red, the other white; **from snow blindness**; sparks in eyes; averse to light; profuse watering after exposure to dry, cold wind; **anxious look**; **burning thirst**.

< fright; **shock**; vexation
< sleeping in sun
< cold, dry wind
< pressure, touch
< noise; light, night
< lying on side; in bed
< music; tobacco smoke

> open air; repose
> warm sweat

Allium cepa

Lachrymation is bland, nasal discharge is irritating (Euph. opposite); much blurring and smarting; **sensitive to light**; eyes suffused and watery; burning of eyelids; hayfever with AM sneezing.

< in evening; warm room	> open air; cold room
	> moving about

Apis (3)

Swollen, red, **edematous** lids; eyes burn and sting; **sudden piercing** pains; **serous exudation**; **suppurative inflammation of eyes**; keratitis with **intense chemosis (edema) of ocular conjunctiva**; profuse hot tears, puffy eyes; photophobia but can't bear covering eyes.

< heat, **room**, weather, drinks	**> cool air**, bathing
< warm bed; hot bath	> uncovering
< touch, even of hair	> slight exertion; motion
< after sleep; 4 PM	
< pressure	

Argentum nit (3)

Inner canthi swollen, **red**; spots before eyes, blurred vision; photophobia in warm room; **purulent ophthalmia**; much swelling of conjunctiva, **much purulent discharge**; unable to keep eyes fixed steadily; aching, tired feeling in eyes > closing or pressing on them; acute granular conjunctivitis, corneal ulcers; **violent pains**, **like deep sticking splinters**; **craves sugar**; **flatulence**; craves fresh air; **thirsty**; chilly.

< emotions, **anxiety**	**> cool air**, bath
< in room; sugar; cold food; on right side	> hard pressure; motion
< looking down; drinking	> eructations
< crowds; night	
< warmth in any form	

Arsenicum alb (3)

Burning eyes with acrid lachrymation, red lids (Sulph), ulcerated, with scabs, scales; edema **around** eyes, painful inflammation,

burning; **hot photophobia**, > external warmth; **restlessness**, **insatiable burning thirst for sips**; **anguish**; **fear of death**.

< cold drinks, foods	**> hot applications, food**, drinks
< cold air	> motion; **elevating head**
< midnight after; 2 AM	> sitting erect; company, sweating
< vegetables, **drinking**	
< eruptions; **exertion**	
< right side	

Belladonna (3)

Dry, injected, painful; **very sensitive to light**; flushed face; overuse; throbbing deep in eyes on lying down; **dilated pupils** (Agnus); eyes feel swollen, protruding, **staring**, **brilliant**; ocular illusions; **diplopia**, squinting, spasm of lids; congested fundus; **restlessness**, lurid, red, terrifying, hallucinations, on closing eyes leading to blind attacks; thirsty.

< heat of sun, if heated	> light covering
< afternoon, 8 PM	> bending backward
< drafts, on head, hair cut	> rest in bed
< washing head, taking cold	> semi-erect
< checked sweat, **light**, **noise**	
< jarring; touch; company	
< pressure; motion; hanging down	

Euphrasia (3)

Lachrymation with irritation due to acrid tears, may have some relief with tearing; **bland discharge from nose**; **eyes constantly water**; **acrid lachrymation**; discharge yellow, thick; burning and swelling of lids; frequent blinking; sticky mucus on cornea, must wink to remove it; pressure in eyes; little blisters on cornea; wants to wipe eyes; coryza is bland (opposite Allium cepa).

< sunlight; **wind**	> open air, winking
< warm room, indoors	> wiping eyes
< evenings, night	> coffee; in dark
< lying down (coryza)	> lying down (cough)

Hepar sulph (2)

Follows Aconite, Belladonna; **very sensitive to cold air**; dry feeling like sand; suppuration; inflammation begins to spread to globe; **very sensitive to any stimulus**; sensation as if eye is being drawn into head; **ulcers on cornea**, purulent conjunctivitis, chemosis (edema), profuse discharge; eyes and lids red, inflamed; eyes sore to touch; bright circles before eyes; boring pain in upper bones of orbit; **chilly and oversensitive**; **sweats easily** with little relief; thirsty;

< **cold**, dry, air, wind, becoming	> **heat**, to head, moist, wraps
< **least uncovering**, **touch**	> **damp weather**
< noise, lying on painful part	> after eating
< night; exertion	

Pulsatilla (2)

Following a cold or flu; not much pain; **thick profuse**, **bland**, **yellow-green discharge**; itching and burning of eyes; **lids inflamed**, **agglutinated**; ophthalmia neonatorum; subacute conditions; **mild weepy**, **emotional**, **changeable**; **shifting symptoms**; craves sympathy; **thirstless**, **peevish**, **chilly**.

< **warmth**, room, air, bed	> **cold**, **fresh air**
< **evenings**, **suppressions**	> uncovering; **erect posture**
< **lying**; **beginning motion**	> gentle motion; continued
< **rich food**, **fats**; **rest**	> crying
< after eating	

Sulphur (3)

Burning ulceration of lid margins; halo around lamp light; heat and **burning in eyes** (Ars,Bell); black spots before eyes; chronic ophthalmia with much burning and itching; cornea like ground glass; yellow discharge with agglutination; follows Aconite; cutting burning pain as if from sand; Sulphur constitutions, **thirsty**; chilly.

< **bathing**; **suppressions**	> open air; motion
< **heated**, milk, **exertion**, **in bed**	> warm applications
< atmosphere changes; speaking	> sweating; **dry heat**

< periodically, 11 AM, full moon	> lying on right side
< rest; standing; alcohol, night	> drawing up affected limbs

Consider:

Calcarea carb (3)

Sensitive to light; lachrymation in open air; early AM; **chronic dilated pupils**; dimness of vision; eyes easily fatigued.

Calcarea sulph (3)

Inflammation of eyes with discharge of thick, **yellow matter**; sees only half an object; corneal ulcers, deep; **thirsty**; chilly.

< drafts, touch	> bathing; open air; eating
< cold; wet; heat of room	> local heat; uncovering

Carboneum sulph (3)

Eye atrophy, impaired vision; color blindness.

Rhus tox (3)

Photophobia, profuse flow of yellow pus; circumscribed corneal injection; corneal ulcers; iritis after exposure to cold; eye painful on turning it or pressing; profuse gush of hot tears with opening eye.

Symptoms in Kent's Repertory	**Page**
Eye, Discharges—see appropriate rubric	237
Eye, Inflammation, infants	242
Eye, Inflammation, conjunctiva	243
Eye, Inflammation, iritis/cornea/canthi	243
Eye, Lachrymation, wind	246
Eye, Pain, warmth agg./amel.	251
Eye, Pain, burning, cold amel.	253
Eye, Pain, burning sand, as if in	254
Eye, Redness, veins	265
Eye, Tears, burning	268
Eye, Ulceration of conjunctiva	269

CONVULSIONS—EPILEPSY—SEIZURES

Convulsions are usually associated with cerebral dysfunction resulting in varying presentations such as slow writhing movements, alternating contraction and relaxation of the muscles, or persistent contraction of the muscles without loss of consciousness. The person may be aware of the impending onset of the seizure or it may develop without warning. Almost any medical condition can lead to convulsions, though in most cases, once the stimulus for it is removed, there will not be a recurrence.

Commonly associated causes are allergens, uremic or toxic poisoning, childbirth, hysteria and hypoglycemia. Brain lesions may be present as a result of these or by themselves.

The important thing to remember when prescribing for this condition is to not panic and to observe carefully what the person is doing as you will obtain many of your symptoms this way. It should also be apparent that this is a very serious condition which needs evaluation by a physician.

Argentum nit (3)

Convulsions without consciousness; **epilepsy**; **epileptiform convulsions**; from fright; during menses; puerperal convulsions; incoordination; loss of balance; **trembling**; sensation as if part were expanding; errors of perception; **time passes slowly**; spots before eyes, blurred vision, photophobia; loss of smell; unconscious passing of urine; cannot walk with eyes closed, trembling and general debility; rigidity of **calves**, debility; walks and stands unsteadily especially when unobserved; numbness of arms; drowsy stupor; ascending paralysis; **violent pains**; **like deeply sticking splinters**; **craves sweets**; faltering speech, gait; epilepsy < night; **flatulence**; peripheral neuralgias; chilly, **thirsty**.

< emotions, anxiety
< in room; **sweets**

> cool, open air
> hard pressure; motion

< lying on right side; looking down
< drinking; crowds
< warmth; at night
< cold foods; **left side**
< menses

> eructations

Baryta carb (2)

Clonic convulsions; epileptic; confusion, senile dementia; alternate dilation and contraction of pupils; sensation of smoke in nose; paralysis of tongue; spasm of esophagus as soon as food enters; numbness of limbs; numb feeling from knees to scrotum; twitching during sleep; heavy pressure over eyes; eyes > looking down, **chilly**, thirsty.

< company, thinking of it
< cold; damp, to feet, head
< lying on left or painful side
< odors; washing

> warm wraps
> walking in open air

Baryta mur (3)

Clonic **epileptic** convulsions; periodic convulsions; **icy coldness of body with paralysis**; **voluntary muscular power gone but perfectly sensible**; whizzing, buzzing in ears; difficulty swallowing; chilly.

Bufo (3)

Convulsions, after anger, begins on abdomen, face; **clonic convulsions**; during coition; **without consciousness**; **epileptic convulsions**, from solar plexus, uterus; epileptiform; from fright; before menses; from suppressed menses; after onanism; from sexual excitement; during sleep; during suppuration; **tonic convulsions**; seizures occur during sleep at night; sensation as if a hot vapor rose to top of head; face bathed in sweat; cannot bear the sight of brilliant objects; disposition to handle genitals, undress (Hyos); **desire for solitude**; trembling, as if electric shocks through body.

< in warm room
< sexual excitement
< during sleep
< least motion; injuries

> bleedings; cool air
> bathing; feet in hot water

Calcarea ars

Epilepsy with rush of blood to head before attack; aura felt in region of heart; flying sensation; anger, anxiety, desires company, great depression; violent rush of blood to head with vertigo; confusion; weariness and lameness of lower limbs; **convulsions from heat** < from slight exertion.

Causticum (3)

Convulsions in AM, evening, night; clonic; from becoming cold; with and without consciousness; **epileptic**, from solar plexus; **epileptiform**; with falling, runs in a circle to fall, from fright, hysterical; **internal convulsions**; before menses, during menses; one-sided convulsions; **with paralysis**, **followed by paralysis**; during sleep; from eruptions; tetanic rigidity; tonic convulsions; progressive loss of muscular strength; local paralysis of vocal cords, muscles of deglutition, tongue, eyelids, face, bladder, extremities; paralysis of right side of face; sparks and dark spots before eyes; **ptosis** (Gels), vision as if a film over eyes; paralysis of ocular muscles after cold exposure; paralysis of single parts, heaviness and weakness, unsteadiness of **muscles of forearms**, hands; loss of sensation in hands, numbness; **contracted tendons**, unsteady walking and falls easily; very drowsy, can hardly keep awake; jerking of single muscles; epilepsy at puberty; **chilly**, **thirsty**.

< dry cold air, **winds**, drafts	**> cold drinks**
< extremes of temperature; stooping	> washing; **warmth** of bed
< coffee; 3–4 AM; **evenings**	> gentle motion
< exertion; suppression; weather changes	**> damp**, **wet weather**
< clear fine weather	
< motion of carriage	

Cicuta virosa (3)

Convulsions in children; **clonic**; from cold air; becoming cold; **without consciousness**; during dentition; spreads downward; epileptic; **epileptiform**, from excitement; falls forward or backward; from fright; during the heat; hysterical convulsions; after injury; during pregnancy; **puerperal**, during sleep; **tetanic rigidity**; **tonic**, **when**

touched; **bends head, neck, and spine backwards**; **violent** action, distortions; moans and howls; sensation of internal chill; delirium with singing, dancing, funny gestures; **one side**; **contracted cervical muscles**; stares persistently at objects; **convulsions** from concussions; **dilated pupils**, **insensible strabismus**, pupils behind upper lids as head inclines; grinds teeth; esophageal spasm, cannot swallow; colic with convulsions; frothing at mouth; tonic spasm of pectoral muscles; curved limbs, cannot be straightened out; suppressed eruptions causes brain disease; prolonged unconsciousness after convulsions; suspicious, childish; turns feet inward or toes up with spasms; thirsty.

< injuries, to brain
< jar; noise; touch
< cold; dentition
< suppressed eruptions
< tobacco smoke; draughts

Cina (3)

At night; from anger **in children**; clonic; **with consciousness**; without consciousness; dentition; epileptic; **epileptiform**; with falling; during heat; internal; after punishment; tonic; **from worms** (Hyos); convulsions with screams and violent jerking of hands and feet; dilated pupils; **pulsation of superciliary muscle**; **choreic movements of face** and hands; **twitching** of limbs; paralyzed shocks, patient jumps suddenly as if in pain; throws arms from side to side; nocturnal convulsions; **sudden inward jerking of fingers of right hand**; **child stretches out feet spasmodically**; left foot in constant spasmodic motion; screams and talks in sleep; ill humor, **very cross**; desires things but rejects what is offered; sensitive to touch; **grinds teeth**, **bluish-white around mouth**; restless sleep; thirsty; **extensor muscles**.

< touch; worms; vexation
< being looked at; full moon
< during sleep; straining; yawning
< in sun; summer

> lying on abdomen; motion
> wiping eyes

Cuprum met (3)

At night; apoplectic; begins in fingers, toes; in children; **clonic**; without consciousness; after coughing; during dentition; **epileptic**; from solar plexus; **epileptiform**; **from eruptions that don't break out**; excitement; **with falling**, forward; from fright; internal; before and during menses; suppressed menses; from metastasis; with paralysis; periodic convulsions; during pregnancy; pressure on stomach; puerperal; during sleep; tetanic; tonic; uremic; **from vexation**; becoming wet; **spasmodic affections**, **cramps**; nausea; epileptic aura begins in knees and spreads to hypogastrium; **thumbs flexed into palms of hands**; child's lips are blue; with consciousness or unconsciousness, foaming and falling; purple, red swelling of head with convulsions; pains increased by movement and touch; eyes are fixed, staring, sunken, glistening, turned upwards; crossed; quick rolling of eyeballs, behind lids; **contraction of jaw**, with foam at mouth; **strong metallic** (Rhus t), **slimy taste**; constant protrusion of tongue like a snake (Lach); stammering speech with long pauses; paralysis of tongue; **contracted** abdomen, colic; **cramps in calves and soles**; weariness of limbs; clenched thumbs, cramps in palms; clonic spasms begin in fingers and toes; shocks in body with sleep; knotting of muscles; twisting of head; exhaustion after contractions; appear to be dead or in a state of ecstasy after the convulsion; cramps in calves > stretching out (opp Calc); fixed ideas, morose, malicious; fearful; uses wrong words; thirsty; spasms **> drinking cold water**, but < cold air; convulsions begin in extremities and work inward; convulsions often begin with a shriek; chorea accompanied by spasmodic vomiting, from fright.

< emotions; anger	> cold drinks
< suppressions; motion	> pressure
< hot weather; vomiting	> during perspiration
< loss of sleep; touch; raising arm	
< before menses; vomiting	

Curare (1)

Epileptic; epileptiform; during heat; tetanic; muscular paralysis without impairing sensation and consciousness; respiratory muscle paralysis; **diminished reflexes**; glycosuria with motor paralysis;

head drawn backward; ptosis of right eye; facial, buccal paralysis, tongue and mouth drawn to right side, red face; **threatened paralysis of respiratory muscles** on falling asleep; **distressing dyspnea**; **arms weak and heavy**; cannot lift fingers; legs tremble and give way, debility, catalepsy.

< dampness; cold weather
< cold wind; 2 AM; right side

Helleborus niger (2)

Convulsions in children; clonic; epileptic; epileptiform; one-sided; puerperal; tetanic; **sensorial depression**; general **muscle weakness**, may go on to paralysis, with dropsical effusions; slow answering, staring, **complete unconsciousness**, **involuntary sighing**; **picks lips and clothes**; **rolls head** day and night; moaning; sudden screams, **bores head into pillow**; cold sweat on forehead; eyeballs turn upward, vacant look, dilated pupils, eyes wide open, sunken; diminished smell; face is pale, sunken, left-sided neuralgia; **falling of lower jaw**, grinds teeth, **chewing motion**; greedily swallows cold water though unconscious; irregular respiration; **automatic motion of one arm and leg**; stretching of limbs; thumb drawn into palm (Cupr); sudden screams in sleep; **criencephaleque**, cannot be fully aroused; lies on back with knees drawn up; gradual onset of advancing weakness; drops things, staggers, won't eat or speak; hydrocephalus; **thirsty**; noise arrests the paroxysm.

< cold air; puberty
< dentition; suppression
< exertion; evening, 4–8 PM
< evening until morning
< uncovering

> strong attention

Hyoscyamus (3)

Night; beings on face; in children, **clonic**, with consciousness; **without consciousness**; coldness; during dentition; after drinking; **epileptic**; **epileptiform**; **from excitement**; **with falling**; from fluids; **from fright**; after grief, after hemorrhage, hysterical; during heat; **internal**; during menses; with paralysis; during pregnancy; **puerperal**, hemorrhage; during sleep, tetanic; tonic; from worms (Cina);

mania of a quarrelsome and obscene character; loquacious; **tremulous weakness and twitching of tendons**; low muttering speech, **constant carphology**, **deep stupor**; dilated pupils, sparkling, fixed; spasmodic closing of lids; objects have colored borders; impaired speech, foams at mouth, lower jaw drops; vomiting with convulsions; involuntary defecation and micturation; **exposes himself** (Bufo); hysterical spasms before menses; spasm of chest forces him to bend forward; epileptic attacks end in deep sleep; cramps in calves and toes; intense sleeplessness, sopor (deep sleep) with convulsions; great restlessness, **every muscle twitches**; doesn't want to be covered; clutching motions; jealous, suspicious, speaks each word louder; averse to light; warm sweat; thirsty.

< emotions, fright, jealousy
< touch; lying; cold, sleep
< at night; menses
< after eating

> sitting up; stooping

Oenanthe crocata (2)

Night; clonic, **coldness of body**; **without consciousness**; **epileptic**; **with falling**; from injuries; before menses; **during menses**; instead of menses; puerperal; tetanic; puerperal eclampsia; uremic convulsions; < pregnancy; **convulsive facial twitching**; pains all over head, dizzy; sudden and complete unconsciousness; furious delirium, giddiness; eyes fixed, dilated pupils; foaming at mouth; lock jaw; much yawning; heavy, spasmodic, stertorous breathing; convulsions, opisthotonus; numbness of hand and foot; cold hands and feet; swollen face; epilepsy, with priapism; status epilepticus.

< injury; menses
< sexual disturbances

Opium (3)

Evening, **night**; after anger; from a bright light; **children**; approach of strangers; **clonic**; coldness of body; without consciousness; epileptic; epileptiform, **from excitement**; with falling, **backwards**; **from fright**; **fright of the mother (infant)**; after grief; during heat; hysterical; from injuries; puerperal; after a shock; during sleep; tetanic; tonic; during vomiting; aggravated by warm bath; drowsy stupor; **painlessness**; **complete loss of consciousness**; **apoplectic state**; delirious talking, with eyes wide open; complete insensibility; eyes half closed, dilated visual hallucinations; pupils insensible, **contracted**; ptosis (Caust, Gels); staring; glassy; face is **swollen**, **dark suffused**, **hot**; besotted look (Bapt, Lach); spasmodic facial twitching, especially corners of mouth; **hanging down of lower jaw**, distorted face; tongue black, **paralyzed**; **intense thirst**; blubbering of lips, difficult articulation and swallowing; opisthotonos; swollen neck veins; painless paralysis (Oleand), **twitching of limbs**; numbness; jerks as if flexors are overacting; convulsions <glare of light; cold limbs; **hot perspiration over whole body except lower limbs**; **placid**, says nothing ails him; heavy, stupid sleep of the aged; not > with perspiration; wants nothing; unable to understand sufferings, lack of will power.

< emotions, **fear**, fright
< odors, **alcohol**, sleep, after sleep
< suppressed discharges
< if heated
< reading, eruptions
< perspiring; brandy, wine
> cold, uncovering
> constant walking
> coffee

Plumbum met (3)

Night, **clonic**; during colic, with consciousness, **without consciousness**; while eating; **epileptic**; **epileptiform**; with falling; hysteria; internal; during menses; after onanism; one-sided; with paralysis; tetany; tonic; uremic; paralysis of extensors, forearm (Curare), upper limbs from center to periphery with partial anesthesia or excessive hyperesthesia, preceded by pain; delirium, coma, convulsions; **progressive muscular atrophy**; infantile paralysis (polio), locomotor ataxia, bulbar paralysis; contractions and boring pains; contracted, yellow pupils; sudden loss of sight after fainting; central scotoma; face **pale and cachectic**, tremor of naso-labial muscles; tongue tremulous, cannot put it out, seems paralyzed; paralysis of lower extremities; paralysis of single muscles; cannot raise or lift anything; difficult extension; pains in muscles of thighs; **come in paroxysms**; **wrist drop**; cramps in calves; stinging, tearing in limbs; twitching and tingling; numbness or tremor; **violent contractions**; chronic epilepsy with marked aura; wasting of paralyzed parts; **naval feels retracted through to spine**; impaired memory, apathy, **fears assassination**; **depression**; thirsty, chilly.

< clear weather; open air	> hard pressure; rubbing
< exertion; motion; company	> hard physical exertion
< grasping smooth objects; touch	> rest, lying down
< night	> stretching limbs

Silicea (2)

Night; children; clonic; with coldness of one side of the body; with and without consciousness; **epileptic**; coldness on left side before epilepsy; sensation like a mouse running before attack; from solar plexus; epileptiform; with falling, forward; internal; after onanism; during sleep; **suppressed foot sweats**; tonic; **after vaccination**; vertigo from looking up; averse to light; cramps in calves and soles; paralytic weakness of forearms; very sensitive to cold, cold air; **very sensitive**; exaggerated reflexes; **foul foot sweats**; **chilly**; profuse **sweat** on upper body; **thirsty**.

< cold air, **draft**, damp	**> warm**, **wraps to head**
< cold bathing, feet; alcohol	> becoming warm
< checked sweat; night; AM	> profuse urination
< mental exertion; light, noise weather	> summer; wet or humid
< jarring of spine; change of motion	
< lying down; lying on left side	

Stramonium (3)

Evening, night; **alternates with excitement of mind, with rage**; apoplectic; **from a bright light**; **changing in character**; **children**; **clonic**, alternates with tonic; from coldness of body; **with consciousness**; without consciousness; during dentition; epileptic; **epileptiform**; exanthema do not appear or are repelled; with falling, backwards; **from fluids**; fright; **during the heat**; hysterical; internal; **aggravated by light**; during menses; after onanism; one sided with paralysis of the other; periodic convulsions; **puerperal**; **from shining objects**; during sleep; suppressed eruptions; secretions and exertions; tonic; when touched; **at the sight of water**; **gyratory**, **graceful motions**; sensation as if limbs separated from body, Parkinson's disease; **raises head frequently from pillow**; **loquacious**; auditory hallucinations; staggers, with tendency to fall forward and to the left; dilated pupils, **staring wide open**, eyes seem prominent, **small objects look large**; facial **expression of terror**; **stammering speech**; risus sardonicus (Nux v), chewing motion; hands constantly on genitals; convulsions after labor (birth); convulsions of upper extremities and isolated muscle groups; chorea, partial spasms, constantly changing; staggering gait; **dreads darkness**; desires company; wants to escape; raving mania; religious insanity; jerks head up then drops it again, sensation of crawling of bugs on body.

< glistening objects; fright	**> light**; company
< after sleep; **dark**, cloudy days	> warmth
< suppressions; intemperance	
< alone; swallowing	

Strychninum (3)

On closing a door; with consciousness; **aggravated by drafts**; epileptic; epileptiform; forcible extension of body ameliorates; tetanic; when touched; stiffness of muscles of neck, face; increased respiration; opisthotonos with convulsions; muscles relax between paroxysm; pains and sensations come **suddenly** and return at **intervals**; restless; **very irritable**; head jerks forward; dilated pupils, sparks before eyes; spasmodic contraction of ocular muscles; twitching; trembling of lids; jaw stiff, spasmodically closed; feces discharged involuntarily with spasms; **spasm of laryngeal muscles**; **rigid cervical muscles**; **stiff back**; violent jerking of spine; **icy sensation down spine**; **violent jerking, twitching and trembling** of extremities; shocks in muscles; **cramp like pains**; consider Nux vomica.

< AM; touch; noise	> lying on back
< motion; after meals	

Consider:

Belladonna (3)

Violent onset, convulsive movements, with high fever; **dilated pupils**; jerking limbs; spasms; **no thirst**, **anxiety or fear**; **in children**; without consciousness; **epileptiform**; **with falling**; **puerperal**; **tonic**.

Calcarea carb (3)

Consider in calcarea constitutions, especially if **convulsions are from fright** or if the **aura spreads from the stomach to the head**.

Cocculus (2)

Painful contracture of trunk and limbs: **trembling** and pain in limbs; limbs straighten out, painful when flexed; epilepsy, epileptiform; **internal**.

Ignatia (2)

Twitching of muscles of face, lips; globus hystericus; jerking of limbs; **hysterical**; **internal**.

Indigo

Epilepsy, with great sadness; undulating sensation through whole head; convulsions; hysterical symptoms; flushes of heat from abdomen to head with epilepsy, fit begins with dizziness; aura from painful spot between shoulders; **from fright**.

Moschus (2)

Fainting fit; convulsions; very sensitive to air, cold; **uncontrollable laughter**; **hysterical** spasm of chest; sudden constriction of larynx, trachea; globus hystericus.

Nux vomica (3)

After anger; **aggravated by drafts**; **from solar plexus**; **during heat**; **internal**, **tetany**.

Platina (1)

Epilepsy; from fright; **after onanism**; **tetany**; **tonic**, **objects look smaller than they are**; hysterical spasms.

Veratrum viride (1)

Twitchings, convulsions; furious delirium, full, **bloated**, **livid face**; convulsive twitching of facial muscles; violent electric-like shocks in limbs.

Zincum met (1)

Weakness, **trembling**, **twitching** of various muscles; **feet in constant motion**; **convulsions with pale face and no heat**; **child repeats everything said to it**; rolls head from side to side; **rolls eyes**; nervous motion when asleep; **in children**; from fright.

Symptoms in Kent's Repertory	**Page**
Eye, Movement, convulsive/rolling	247
Back, Opisthotonos	893
Generals, Convulsions, children	1352
Generals, Convulsions, consciousness, with	1352
Generals, Convulsions, dentition, during	1352
Generals, Convulsions, fright, from	1354
Generals, Convulsions, injuries, from	1354
Generals, Convulsions, paralysis, with	1354
Generals, Convulsions, shining objects from	1355
Generals, Convulsions, tetanic rigidity	1355
Generals, Convulsions, vaccination, after	1356
Generals, Convulsions, worms, from	1356

CROUP

Most often seen in young children, **croup** is characterized by a labored and suffocative breathing, persistent and troublesome cough, and is associated with laryngeal spasm or a membranous deposit on the larynx. The **cough** often has a characteristic metallic ring to it and comes in waves or recurring suddenly with an intensifying of symptoms. Breathing may show an irregular bumpy-like rhythm termed "stridor," and the person may appear quite anxious, fearful or panicked.

Croup has been associated with **membranous diphtheria**, a disease not seen as much today as in the early years of this century. However, it can cause a closing-off of the larynx. This, of course, is a medical emergency and needs to be evaluated by a physician.

Aconite (3)

Sudden onset; **oppressed breathing** on least motion; **hoarse**, **dry**, **croupy cough**; loud labored breathing; child grasps at throat with every cough; sensitive to inspired air; **shortness of breath**; cough, dry, short, hacking; **< at night and after midnight**; hot feeling in lung; chest tingles after cough; sensitive larynx; stitches in chest; sits erect with cough; ringing, whistling cough; cough is < drinking; fever; **dry hot skin**; **high fever**; look of **terror**, **anxiety**, **fear**; very **restless**, **burning thirst**; fears death; part of the Aconite-Spongia-Hepar triad.

< fright, **shock**
< sleeping in sun
< cold, dry winds, sweating
< pressure; touch
< noise; light, during menses
< during dentition; night; in bed
< lying on side; warm room
< music; tobacco smoke

> open air; repose
> warm sweat

Belladonna (2)

Dryness of nose, fauces, larynx and trachea; **tickling**, **short**, **dry cough**; **cough < night**; larynx feels sore; oppressed respiration, quick, unequal; **hoarse**, loss of voice; painless hoarseness; cough with pain in left hip; **barking cough**, whooping cough, with pain in stomach before attack; bloody expectoration; stitches in chest with coughing; **larynx very painful**, feels as if a foreign body were in it; **high piping voice**; **moaning at every breath**, **sudden onset**; **delirious**; **throbbing**, face hot and dry, flushed but sweating on covered parts; drinks in sips; **photophobia**; **dilated pupils**; urging to swallow with choking; **bright red**, **glossy skin**; cries out suddenly; **no thirst**, **anxiety or fear**; thirsty.

< heat, of sun; afternoon (3 PM)
< drafts, on head; hair cut
< washing head; taking cold
< checked sweat; **light**; **noise**
< jarring; touch; pressure
< company; motion; hanging down

> bending backward
> bed rest; light covering
> semi erect

Bromium (2)

Dry cough with hoarseness, burning pain **behind sternum**; **spasmodic cough with rattling of mucus** in larynx; **hoarseness**; suffocative; **croup** after febrile symptoms have subsided; difficult and painful breathing; violent cramping of chest; chest pains run upward; **cold sensation with inspiration**; inspiration provokes cough; **laryngeal diphtheria**; membrane begins in larynx and spreads upward; difficulty getting air into lungs; asthma; bronchial tubes feel filled with smoke; inhaled air feels smoky, raw or cold; wants to take a deep breath but it causes a cough; suffocative fits, starts up choked with croupy or wheezing cough or with palpitation; spasm of glottis; asthma of sailors going ashore; hoarseness < if heated; **blonde children**; profuse sweats, great weakness; chilly.

< warm; **dampness**; overheating
< chilled while hot
< sea breathing; lying on left side
< dust; drafts
< until midnight

> nosebleeds; at sea
> motion; exercise

Drosera (1)

Fits of deep, barking or choking cough; incessant cough which comes from the abdomen and may cause difficulty in catching their breath; person **holds sides** from the soreness from prolonged coughing; cough followed by retching or vomiting; **coughing fits follow in rapid succession** making it difficult for the person to breathe which may lead to convulsions; **hoarse cough, voice**; ***cough with lying down at night but not during the day;*** voice is hollow, toneless; laryngitis, sore throats from speaking; scraping, rough feeling in the upper throat and larynx, sensation of a constant tickle or feather in throat; sense of constriction, stitching pains in chest which is < talking; asthma, whooping cough, colds which settle in the throat and eyes; effects of exposure to cold damp (Dulc), air conditioning; nose bleeds, cold sweats may accompany illness.

< lying down
< midnight, after midnight, 2 AM
< talking, laughing
< cold food and drink

Hepar sulph (3)

Exposure to dry, cold wind, loses voice, coughs; hoarseness; dry, hoarse cough; cough with walking; cough excited **whenever any part of the body gets cold or uncovered**, or from eating anything cold; croup with loose rattling cough; **choking cough**; rattling, croaking cough; suffocative attacks, has to rise up and bend head backwards; anxious wheezing, moist breathing; asthma < in dry, cold air, > damp; painful larynx; **loose** cough but can't expectorate; **weakness and much rattling in chest**; much expectoration, thick, yellow; skin sensitive, to cold air; **chilly**, **oversensitive**; **sticking** splinter like pains; **sweats easily**; irritable; dissatisfied; bad temper; thirsty, hasty speech; part of Aconite-Spongia-Hepar triad.

< cold dry **air, winter, drafts**
< lying on painful part
< parts becoming cold
< least, uncovering; touch
< exertion; night; noise

> heat; warm wraps to head
> moist heat
> damp weather
> after eating

Iodum (3)

Raw, tickling sensation which provokes a dry cough; **pain in larynx**; hoarseness; child grasps throat when coughing; internal dry heat, external coldness; difficult expansion of chest; blood streaked sputum; croup in scrofulous children with dark hair and eyes; inspiration difficult; dry morning cough, from tickling in larynx; **croupy cough , downward from head to throat and bronchi**; weakness of chest; tickling all over chest; rough voice; short of breath; cough < indoors, warm wet weather, lying on back, **cross**, **restless**; **hard**, **swollen glands**; **always too hot**; patient will throw back their head and/ or grasp larynx in order to get air; symptoms are often < in AM; **thirsty**.

< heat, **room**, air, wraps	**> cold**, **air**, breathing
< exertion, ascending, talking	> motion, eating; open air
< fasting; night; rest	
< quiet; right side	

Ipecac—See **Asthma**.

Kali bic (3)

Voice hoarse, < evening; metallic, hacking cough; **profuse**, **yellow expectoration**, **very glutinous and sticky**, comes out in **long**, **stringy and very tenacious** mass; tickling in larynx; true membranous croup, extending to larynx and nares; cough with pain in sternum, extends to shoulders; lumpy, thick discharges; tickling cough after eating, with eructations; heart feels weak, cold; **chilly**, thirsty.

< cold, **air**, water, draft	> warmth; sitting with elbows on knees
< hot weather	> open air
< 2–3 AM; winter	
< overheating; beer	
< lying on left or painful side	
< undressing (cough); eating	

Lachesis (2)

Upper part of windpipe very susceptible to touch; sensation of suffocation and strangulation on lying down, especially **when any-**

thing is around throat; patient springs from bed and rushes to open window; spasm of glottis; feels as if something ran from neck to larynx; **feels he must take a deep breath**; cough, dry, suffocative fits, tickling; little secretion and much sensitiveness; **breathing almost stops on falling asleep** (Grind); larynx painful to touch; sensation of a plug (Anac)which moves up and down, with a short cough; cough < touching neck or auditory canal, > with expectoration; air hunger; **excessive painfulness of throat**; **symptoms move from left to right**; **loquacious**; fears going to sleep; thirsty but fears to drink; restless; suspicious; chilly.

< sleep, **after**, AM
< heat, **summer**, **sun**, **room**
< warm drinks;
< swallowing liquids; left side
< slight touch; **pressure**
< retarded discharges; **alcohol**
< start and close of menses
< cloudy weather; **empty swallowing**
< closing eyes

> open air; **discharges**
> hard pressure; bathing part
> cold drinks
> warm applications

Phosphorus (3)

Hoarseness, < evenings, **larynx very painful**; **cannot talk due to pain in larynx**; cough from tickling in throat; **< cold air**, **talking**; sweet taste while coughing; hard, dry, tight, racking cough; cough from going from warm room into cold air; **tightness across chest**; **great weight on chest**; whole body **trembles** with cough; pain in throat on coughing; nervous cough; blood streaked sputum; emptiness in chest; **craves cold drinks**; croupy, then bronchitis; cough exhausts; **chilly**; **suddenness of symptoms**; very sensitive.

< lying on left, painful side
< emotions; talking; touch; odors
< light; puberty
< lying on back
< cold, **hands**, open air
< warm ingesta; salt
< sexual excesses
< weather changes; windy

> eating; sleep
> cold, food, water to face
> being rubbed
> sitting up
> in dark; lying on right side

< AM and evenings; mental fatigue
< ascending stairs

Sambucus (3)

Spasmodic croup; paroxysmal, **suffocative cough**, **coming on about midnight**, with crying and dyspnea; hoarseness with tenacious mucus in larynx; oppression of chest with pressure in stomach, nausea; **sniffles in infants**; dry coryza; loose choking cough;**child awakes suddenly**, **nearly suffocating**, **sits up**, **turns blue**; **cannot expire** (Mephitis); **sudden suffocation**; strangling cough on falling asleep; whistling breathing; spasm of glottis; screeching voice; dry burning heat during sleep but copious sweat on waking; **profuse sweat** with cough;**constant fretfulness**; easily frightened; thirstless.

< dry, cold air
< cold drinks; while heated
< head low; sleep
< during rest; after eating fruit

> pressure over a sharp edge
> motion; wrapping up
> sitting up in bed

Spongia (3)

Great dryness of air passages; **hoarseness**, **larynx dry**, **burns**, **constricted**; cough **dry**, **barking**, **croupy**; larynx sensitive to touch; **croup**, **< inspiration and before midnight**; short, panting, **difficult** respiration; **sensation of a plug in larynx**; **cough abates after eating or drinking**, especially warm drinks; irrepressible cough from a spot deep in chest, raw and sore; oppression and heat of chest; with sudden weakness; asthma with profuse expectoration and **suffocation**; **hollow cough**; choking on falling asleep; terrified, anxious, cough from excitement.

< dry, **cold** wind
< roused from sleep
< exertion; raising arms
< before 12 midnight
< ascending

> eating a little
> head lying low
> descending

Consider:

Phytolacca (2)

Difficulty breathing; dry, hacking, tickling cough, < midnight; aching pain in chest; through mid—sternum, with cough; indifferent to life; **sore**, **hard ache** all over; restlessness; < cold, damp,> warm, dry.

Rumex (2)

Tickling in throat pit causes cough; **copious mucous discharge** from nose, trachea, **dry**, **teasing cough preventing sleep**; **cough aggravated by pressure**, **talking**; **inspiration of cool air**, **at night**; rawness of larynx and trachea; **raw pain under clavicle** , soreness only behind sternum, especially left side; dry, sensitive mucous membranes; **continuous cough**; frothy expectoration, < cool air, pressure on trachea, uncovering; > covering mouth, wrapping up; chilly.

Stramonium

Raises head frequently from pillow: expression of terror; pale face or red, hot; cannot swallow due to spasm; awakens terrified; screams with fright; **dreads darkness**; spasmodic cough; spasm of larynx; < alone, on swallowing; > company, warmth.

Sulphur

Oppression, burning in chest; **difficult respiration**, **wants windows open**; loose cough; **dyspnea** in middle of night, > sitting up; **much rattling of mucus**; heat throughout chest; < heated, bathing; > open air, warm applications.

Symptoms in Kent's Repertory	**Page**
Cough, Night/various times	780
Cough, Air, cold	781
Cough, Air, open/amel	782
Cough, Barking	782
Cough, Choking	783
Cough, Constriction, larynx	784
Cough, Croupy	785

See rubrics under **Bronchitis** for chest pains associated with coughs.

CYSTITIS—INFLAMMATION OF BLADDER

Cystitis is an inflammation of the bladder and/or urethra. More commonly found in women, there are a number of predisposing factors which lead to bacterial infection. Among them are irritation from sexual intercourse, poor hygiene, obstruction by an enlarged prostate gland, chemical irritants, variations in estrogen levels and venereal diseases, to name a few.

Symptoms of frequent and intense desire to urinate are accompanied by burning with the passing of urine. Tenderness over the bladder, a slight fever and an increased thirst may be present as well. The urine itself may be very bloody in appearance and possess a strong odor. Careful notation of the objective (what you observe) and subjective (what the person tells you) symptoms are important for good prescribing.

While bacteria are present with cystitis, they are not really the cause of the condition. Bacterial organisms are normally found in close proximity to the male and female urethra, and it is the body's ability to resist their spread that keeps an infection from occurring. An infection that is not treated or does not respond fully to therapy is at risk for developing into a **kidney infection** and needs to be evaluated by a physician.

Aconite (3)

Scanty, **red**, **hot**, **painful** urination; tenesmus and burning at neck of bladder; urethral burning; suppressed urine; **retention with screaming and restlessness**; handles genitals; anxiety with beginning to urinate; profuse urination with profuse perspiration and diarrhea; **much fear**; **restless**, **burning thirst**.

< fright, shock	> open air; repose
< cold dry winds	> warm sweat
< pressure, touch	

< noise, light; menses
< warm room
< night; on affected side

Apis (3)

Burning, soreness with urination; suppressed urine; casts in urine; frequent, involuntary urination; stinging pain and painful urination (strangury); **scanty high colored urine**; incontinence; **last drops burn** and **smart**; foul smelling urine; coffee ground sediment; nephritis; thirstless.

< heat; touch, pressure
< late afternoon; after sleep
< closed, heated room
< right side
< warm drinks

> open air; uncovering
> cold bathing
> motion

Benzoic acid

Cystitis, nephritis; uric acid diathesis; pain between urination; urine smells like horse urine; dark brown urine; **repulsive odor**; **enuresis**; **dribbling** offensive urine in old men; hot urine.

< open air; cold
< weather changes

> urination
> heat

Cannabis indica (2)

Slimy mucous in urine; strains, **dribbling**; waits for urine to flow; dull pain region of right kidney.

Cannabis sativa (1)

Pain at beginning of urination which stops by the time flow ceases; **pain from urethra to bladder**; urination difficult to start; dribbling; split stream; inflamed sensation; sore to touch; urine scalds, spasmodic closure of sphincter; acute stage of gonorrhea; walks with legs apart; zigzag pain along urethra; urethral caruncle (Eucalyptus); phimosis; stoppage of urethra by mucus and pus; **scanty burning urine passed drop by drop**; priapism; **ideation and perception exalted**, **mental excitement**.

< darkness; urinating
< exertion, talking, walking
< lying down; gonorrhea

Cantharis (3)

Intolerable urging and tenesmus; severe pain, stinging, cutting, burning; bloody urine by drops; pain before, during and after urine; **urine scalds**, is **passed drop by drop**; **constant desire to urinate**; urine jelly-like; cystitis goes into nephritis; dread of urinating; may or may not have a fever; thirst.

< taking cold; lifting
< after menses; shaving
< touch; urinating
< drinking cold water, coffee

> continued motion
> rubbing

Causticum (2)

Pain with urination; burning; cutting; severe progressive pain; loss of urine with cough (Puls); expels urine slowly; involuntary loss with first sleep; **retention** after surgery; loss of sensibility on passing urine; **thirsty**; **chilly**.

< exertion
< dry, cold winds
< clear weather
< motion of car
< 3–4 AM, evening
< stooping
< weather changes

> damp wet weather
> warmth, gentle motion

Equisetum (3)

Frequent urging with **severe pain at close of urination**; severe dull pain; feeling of fullness in bladder not relieved by urinating; urine flows drop by drop; may have increased urine flow with cystitis; sharp **burning**, cutting pains in urethra while urinating; incontinence in children, elderly; retention and dysuria during pregnancy and after delivery; much mucus in urine; albuminuria; **nocturnal enuresis**; irritable bladder.

< at close of urination	> in afternoon
< pressure; movement	> lying down
< right side	
< sitting down	

Lycopodium (3)

Pain in back before urinating which ceases after flow; **urine slow to start**, straining; retention of urine; **polyuria during the night**; **heavy red sediment**; child cries before urinating (Bor); frequent urging especially from riding; acrid urine; scanty; thirstless; chilly.

< pressure of clothes	> warm drinks, food
< warmth; awakening; wind	> cold applications
< 4–8 PM; indigestion	> motion; eructations
	> urinating
	> after midnight
	thirst & stomach > warmth

Mercurius cor

Continuous passing of blood; **painful tenesmus**; **passes urine in small amounts**; hot, burning; scanty or suppressed urine; **bloody greenish discharge**; **albumin in urine**; perspiration after urinating; pain from urethra to bladder; thirsty.

< urinating, stool	> rest
< swallowing	
< night; cold; autumn	
< hot damp; cool nights	
< acids	

Pulsatilla (3)

Burning, stitching pain during & after urination; profuse urine; increased desire; **< with lying down**; burning at orifice; involuntary loss with coughing (Caust), passing flatus; spasmodic pain in bladder; **dry mouth**; **no thirst**; common remedy with *E. coli* infection.

< heat; fats; eating	**> open air**; motion
< spicy foods, warm room	> cold applications
< evenings	

< lying on left or painless side
< feet hanging down

Sarsaparilla (3)

Severe pain at conclusion of urination; **urine dribbles while sitting**; ineffectual urging; bladder distended; tender; **passes urine only while standing**; urine scanty; slimy, sandy, **bloody**; renal colic, kidney stones; **pain from right kidney downward**; tenesmus of bladder; pain at meatus; pain causes patient to scream; gassy urine; moist, foul genitals.

< after urinating
< spring; cold; wet
< night; yawning
< before menses

> uncovering neck or chest
> standing

Sepia (3)

Thick, foul urine; **red, adhesive sand**; involuntary urination **during first sleep**; chronic cystitis; slow urination; bearing down sensation in pelvis; thirstless; chilly.

< cold air, wet
< sexual excesses
< before menses
< pregnancy, abortion
< AM & PM; after first sleep
< dampness; left side
< before thunderstorms

> violent motion
> warmth
> cold drinks; bathing
> drawing limbs up
> after sleep

Staphysagria (2)

Honeymoon cystitis, **following sexual relations**, **after physical or sexual abuse**; ineffectual urging to urinate; cystitis in lying in patients; bladder feels as if it didn't empty, pressure; **cystocele**; **sensation as if a drop of urine were continually rolling along the channel**; burning in urethra with and without urinating; frequent urination; urging and pain after urination; pain after lithotomy; increased sexual desire; prostatitis; nervous; irritable; urinates in a slender stream; thirstless; chilly.

< anger, indignation, grief
< mortification; tobacco
< sexual excesses, loss of fluids
< masturbation
< touch on affected parts
< cold drinks
< night

> warmth, rest

Terebinthina (3)

Strangury with bloody urine; scanty, suppressed urine; **odor of violets**; urethritis with painful erections; inflamed kidneys following any acute disease; constant tenesmus; nephritis; cystitis, pains alternate between bladder and navel; urine smoky, muddy, yellow, thick secretions; dark black urine—consider if Merc doesn't work.

< dampness; cold; night
< lying; pressure

> motion

Consider:

Arsenicum alb

Low urinary output with **burning pains** and involuntary loss of urine; **albumin in the urine**; sediment contains much mucus, epithelial cells, pus and blood; good remedy for glomerular nephritis; feeling of weakness following urination.

Berberis

Urine has a **thick**, **bright red** (Lyc) and mealy (powder-like) sediment; sensation as if urine remained after urination; **pain in the region of the thighs and loins with urination**; stitching pains which run from the kidneys to the bladder with or without urination; good remedy for colic from passage of stones.

Capsicum

Intense burning of the urethral orifice; urinary flow comes in drops then spurts; spasm of the urethral orifice which allows for a hesitating and painful flow of urine; frequency, ineffectual urging.

Nux vomica

Frequency and **urging but is unable to pass urine** or passes a little at a time; itching in urethra with urination; pain spreads from kidneys to urethra; spasm of the urethra.

Sabina

Urging; inflammation with much throbbing in bladder and kidneys; **bright, red blood from urethra, with clots; pain extends from sacrum to pubic bone.**

Uva ursi

Cystitis, with pain, spasm and mucus discharge with urination; **intense burning after passing of a thick and slimy urine**; frequent urging with burning and tearing pains; sediment contains many WBCs, RBCs and a thick, tenacious mucus which is passed in large masses or clots; good for **pyelonephritis**, infection due to stones and for chronic vesicle irritation.

Auto nosode—Auto nosodes (a remedy which is made from a product of the disease from the patient), work well in cases of chronic urinary tract infections due to urethral reflux or in cases of chronic indwelling catheters. They can be prepared by culturing and isolating the infecting organism. You can use either an alcohol extraction or cut with lactose, and follow the procedure for preparation of dilutions and succussion. Several homeopathic pharmacies have nosode preparations available of the more common infecting organisms, or you can contact them and they will prepare them for you. I have seen them work well in low potencies, 6x to 30c.

Symptoms in Kent's Repertory	Page
Bladder, Inflammation, neck	646
Bladder, Pain, urinating, beginning	647
Bladder, Pain, urinating, during	649
Bladder, Retention, in children	650
Bladder, Retention, painful	651
Bladder, Urging, painful	654

DIARRHEA—CHILDREN

Diarrhea has a number of causes and is seen as an attempt by the body to eliminate some form of toxic or harmful agent. Most everyone will suffer from an acute diarrhea at one time or another, which usually is self-limiting. In infants and children, however, the condition can become quite severe, resulting in a loss of fluids and electrolytes which leads to dehydration. This condition can develop quite rapidly, and supervision by a physician and/or hospitalization is necessary.

Children's diarrhea is quite often associated with intolerance to formula feeding, milk or wheat. Introduction of foods too soon before the digestive system has had time to develop predisposes infants to chronic diarrhea and food intolerances.

Chronic diarrhea usually indicates a serious underlying condition such as colitis, gastritis, parasite infection, heavy metal toxicity, infected water supply or a reaction to anxiety, stress or fear. Cases lasting over 72 hours or which lead to a rapid dehydration and extreme fatigue need to be evaluated by a physician. As with acute diarrhea, fluid and electrolyte loss also need to be considered when evaluating someone with chronic diarrhea.

Aconite (2)

Watery diarrhea; frequent small stool with tenesmus; **green, like chopped herbs**; abdomen is **sensitive to touch**; burning in umbilical region; comes on after exposure to cold dry wind; **great fear, anxiety**; **fears future, restlessness**; impatient, anxious; **burning thirst**; abdominal symptoms > after warm soup; bloody stools; **thirsty**.

< violent emotions, fright	> open air
< sleeping in sun	> warm sweat
< cold, dry winds; sweating	> repose
< pressure, touch	

< noise, light, dentition
< night; lying on affected side
< warm rooms; tobacco smoke

Aethusa (3)

Stool **undigested, thin, greenish**; colic and tenesmus before stool followed by exhaustion and drowsiness; cholera infantum; bubbling sensation around navel; cold internal and external; aching pain in bowels; **intolerance of milk**; nausea at sight of food; violent onsets, exhaustion and lack of reaction; convulsions; some thirst.

< milk; dentition	> open air, company
< hot weather; summer	
< frequent eating	
< over exertion	
< 3–4 AM; evenings	

Arsenicum alb (2)

Diarrhea from spoiled food; too much fruit; **frequent dark offensive stools, restlessness**; thirst for small sips of water; **weakness and prostration**; cholera with intense agony, prostration and burning thirst; body is ice cold (Verat); **great fear**; foul rice water or small, acrid, lienteric stools; **much thirst, chilly**.

< cold, drinks; food	**> hot applications, food, drink**
< cold air	
< periodically, midnight	> motion
< after 2 AM, every 14 days, yearly	**> elevating head**
< vegetables, drinking	> sitting erect, company
< infections, eruptions	> sweating
< lying on part; tobacco	
< exertion	

Calcarea carb (3)

Diarrhea of undigested food, fetid with ravenous appetite; **children's diarrhea**; constipation with hard stool (Bry) then pasty then liquid; chalky gray or green watery stools; lienteric stools; **enlarged glands**; **dilated pupils**; milk aggravates; **thirst** for cold drinks, **chilly**.

< cold, **air**, **bathing**
< weather changes
< exertion of any type
< dentition; puberty
< pressure of clothes
< milk, awaking, anxiety
< ascending; full moon
< wet weather

> dry climate, weather
> lying on painful side

Chamomilla (3)

Greenish slimy stools with teething; hot, **green**, watery, fetid, slimy stools with colic; **chopped white and yellow mucous like chopped egg and spinach**; anus is sore; flatulent colic after anger; **red cheeks and hot perspiration**; irritable; **oversensitive**; **cross**, **ugly**; **quarrelsome**; **wants to be carried**; **lienteric stools** smell like bad eggs; hot and thirsty.

< anger, **night**, **teething**
< cold, air, damp, wind
< coffee; narcotics; alcohol

> being carried
> mild weather; heat
> sweating
> cold applications
> warm wet weather

Colocynthis

Severe cramping, **patient bends double**; rush of diarrhea; **dysenteric stool comes on each time by the least food or drink**; **jelly-like stools**; musty odor; yellow frothy watery, shreddy, sourish stools; colic and gas; slippery bubbles escape from anus; anger, easily vexed, thirsty.

< emotions, **vexation**
< lying on painless side
< night, in bed; drafts
< taking cold, indignation

> hard pressure
> coffee; heat; rest
> gentle motion
> after stool or flatus
> doubling up

Ipecac (3)

Amoebic dysentery with tenesmus; **pain worse around navel**; stools pitch like, **green**, **like frothy molasses**; slimy stools; bloody stool; **no thirst**; balls of mucus in stool; **continuous nausea**; vomiting may or may not be present; chilly.

< warmth; damp, room	> open air
< overeating; veal	
< periodically; heat and cold	
< moist warm wind	
< lying down	

Magnesia carb (2)

Rumbling, gurgling of abdomen; pain in right iliac region; stool preceded by griping colicky pain; **green**, **water**, **frothy like frog pond scum**; bloody mucous filled stools; **undigested milk in nursing children**; lienteric, gelatinous masses in stool; **sour-smelling stool**, with tenesmus (Rheum), thirsty; chilly.

< night; rest, noise	> motion
< cold, wind, drafts	> open air, warm air
< weather changes	
< food, starchy, milk	
< touch, slightest cause	
< warmth of bed; rest	
< every three weeks	

Magnesia mur (3)

Constipation of infants during dentition.

Mercurius (3)

Greenish, **bloody and slimy stools < at night**; **pain and tenesmus**; **never get done sensation**; whitish-grey stools; scanty stools; swollen inguinals; weakened bowels; **easy profuse sweat**; **much prostration**; extremes of temperature bothers them; **extreme thirst**, chilly.

< night; **sweating**; **heated** from bed	> moderate temperature
< lying on right side	
< drafts to head	
< cloudy, cold damp weather	
< heat and cold	

< wet feet; firelight
< weather changes

Natrum sulph

Burning in abdomen and anus; **bruised sensation with pain and urging to stool**; **diarrhea is yellow**, **watery**; **loose stools in AM**; **flatulence**, < before breakfast; colic in ascending colon; < after a spell of wet weather; involuntary passage of stool with flatus; **large fecal mass expelled**; **rumbling**, **gurgling in bowels then sudden gurgling**, **noisy**, **sputtering stool**; stool drives him from bed in AM (Sulph, Bry), yellow diarrhea, foamy, mixed with green slime; sensitive; **feels every weather change**; thirsty.

< lying on left side; touch
< head injuries; lifting
< pressure; late evenings, wind; light; music
< diarrhea
< cold drinks, farinaceous food, vegetables, cold evening air

> position changes
> dry weather

Nux vomica

Diarrhea from overfeeding; stool passed with difficulty in small amounts; **stool relieves pain for a while**; sensation as if some left in rectum; thirsty, **chilly**.

< early AM, **cold**, **uncovering**
< open air, sedentary
< fatigue; disturbed sleep
< slightest noise, odors, touch
< pressure of clothes; anger

> free discharges
> naps, **resting**
> wrapping head, hot drinks
> milk; moist air

Podophyllum (3)

Green, watery, undigested food forcibly expelled most often in morning; **profuse**, **purulent**, **putrid**, **projectile**, prolapse of rectum before or with stool; diarrhea of long standing, **4 AM diarrhea**; **during teething with hot glowing cheeks**; diarrhea in hot weather after acid fruits; while being waked or bathed; cholera infantum and morbus; **stools gush painlessly**; summer diarrheas; stools cornmeal mush-like or in lumps like milky-colored chalk; diarrhea alternates with constipation (Ant c); thirsty.

< early AM; eating
< hot weather; dentition
< drinking; motion

> stroking liver
> lying on abdomen

Psorinum (3)

Stool with **bloody mucus, excessively fetid, dark fluid**; penetrating odor to stool; cholera infantum; **hungry** or unusually well **before an attack**; **anxiety**; scruffy dirty looking children; dreads cold drafts; some thirst, **chilly**.

< cold; open air, weather
< stormy, changing weather
< heat; of bed, exertion
< suppressions; coffee
< contact of his own limbs

> lying quietly with head low
> eating, washing
> nosebleeds; hard pressure
> profuse sweating

Rheum (3)

Sour diarrhea, **whole child smells sour:** unsuccessful urging to urinate before stool; pasty stools; shivering, tenesmus and burning of anus with stool; ineffectual urging to stool; impatient children always crying or screaming; stool brown, green, fermented slimy, acrid, sour: stool > eating unripe fruit.

< dentition; eating; summer
< uncovering; moving about

> warmth; wrapping up

Stramonium (3)

Putrid, dark, painless, involuntary diarrhea; dry throat with great thirst yet dreads water; **dread of darkness**; **night terrors, child strikes or bites**; **very irritable**.

< glistening objects, fright
< after sleep
< dark, cloudy days
< dark room; alone
< swallowing; suppressions

> light; company
> warmth

Sulphur (3)

Morning diarrhea, painless and drives patient out of bed; prolapse of rectum; changing, mushy, stinking, watery, gray froth, < milk diarrhea; alternates with constipation; 5 AM diarrhea (Phos); thirsty, chilly.

< **suppressions**; **bathing**	> open air; motion
< heated, in bed, exertion	> warm applications
< atmospheric changes	> sweating; lying on right side
< speaking; 11 AM; full moon	> dry heat
< rest	> drawing up affected limbs

Symptoms in Kent's Repertory	**Page**
Rectum, Diarrhea, driving out of bed	609
Rectum, Diarrhea, rising, after	609
Rectum, Diarrhea, waking with urging	610
Rectum, Diarrhea, children, in	611
Rectum, Diarrhea, dentition, during	612
Rectum, Diarrhea, drinking water, from	612
Rectum, Diarrhea, milk, after	614
Rectum, Flatus, diarrhea, during	617
Rectum, Involuntary, stool, flatus, passing	621
Rectum, Pain, diarrhea, during	625
Stool, Forcible	637
Stool, Mucus, bloody	639
Stool, Thin, liquid, pouring out	642
Generalities, Emaciation, loss of fluids	1358
Generalities, Weakness, diarrhea	1416

DYSMENORRHEA

Dysmenorrhea is a condition of difficult and painful menstrual flow which may have a variety of causes. It is to be distinguished from the premenstrual syndrome which also has some of the same symptomatology. Often the two are indistinguishable from one another, as both conditions are characterized by painful cramping, irritability and fatigue.

Symptoms are caused by an imbalance between the estrogen and progesterone ratios of the female menstrual cycle. Once this imbalance is corrected, a normal flow resumes. Persistent symptoms of dysmenorrhea may also be an indication of an ovarian cyst, cervical dysplasia or endometriosis, all potentially serious conditions.

Belladonna (3)

Congestion, **sensation of heaviness in abdomen**, **of bearing down**; hot, warm pelvis; much menses, bright red, early, profuse; menses and lochia offensive, hot; cutting pain from hip to hip (Cimic); **restless**; **head sensitive to drafts**; bearing-down sensation> standing < lying; cramps extending from uterus to back, provoked by dark, almost black blood with clots; thirst and thirstless.

< heat, of sun
< afternoon (3 PM)
< drafts; haircut
< washing head; taking cold
< checked sweat; **light**; **noise**
< jarring; touch; company
< motion; pressure

> semi erect
> light covering
> bending backward
> rest in bed

Borax (2)

Membranes and tissue pass with menses; **early**, **profuse** with colic and nausea; pruritus of vulva, eczema, sensation of distended clitoris; pain of menses with griping, nausea and stomach pain extending to small of back; **fears downward motion**; starts at trifles, **dry skin**, averse to coition, thirsty.

< downward motion	> 11 PM; pressure
< sudden noises; cold	> cold weather
< least uncovering, fruit	
< children; smoking	
< warm weather	

Bryonia (1)

Vicarious menses, with nose bleeds rather than flow; headache with menses; associated gastric symptoms with menses; **inter-menses pains with much abdominal and pelvic soreness** (Ham); stitching pain in ovaries with deep inspiration; sensitive to light touch; **averse to least motion**; **thirst for large drinks**; heavy, hard breasts before menses; pain in right ovary, extending to thigh (Lilium, Croc).

< motion, any	**> pressure**, **lying on painful side**
< warm weather	**> cool open air**, **guilt**
< dry heat, cold	> cloudy, damp days
< hot, **becoming**, room,	> drawing knees up
< eating, **vexation**	> heat to inflamed parts
< touch, early AM	**> rest**
< suppressions, taking cold	

Cactus grand (3)

Constricting pain, grabbing; patient cries out; pulsating pains of uterus; early menses; dark, pitch-like (Cocc, Mag c), cease on lying down; with cardiac symptoms; vaginismus, **hemorrhages**.

< lying on left side, occiput	> open air
< exertion; night	> pressure on vertex
< periodically, 10–11 AM or PM	

Calcarea phos (3)

Menses early, excessive, bright red, is dark red if late; bright red to dark red with **violent backache**; nymphomania (Plat), with aching, pressing or weakness in uterine region; uterus heavy, weak; menses every 2 weeks; **chilly**.

< weather changes, drafts	> lying down
< cold, wet, east wind	
< mental exertion; loss of fluids	
< puberty	

Caulophyllum (2)

Dull, drowsy, droopy (Gels), congestion; feels weak and trembly, scanty flow; sensation of a weight in uterus; pains travel all directions; needle like pains; profuse menses; spasmodic, severe pains; aborts easily; menses and leukorrhea profuse; **erratic pains**, drawing pains; vomiting from uterine pain; fretful, fearful, chilly.

< pregnancy, suppressed menses
< open air
< PM

Chamomilla (3)

Profuse discharge of **dark clotted blood with labor-like pains**; spasmodic pains; pains press upward (Gels), cannot stand pains (Caul, Caust, Gels, Hyos, Puls); oversensitive; **irritable**, **ugly**, **cross**, **quarrelsome**, dark lumpy menses or lochia; pains go up and down thighs; sharp pains to numbness; **thirsty**.

< anger; **night**	> mild weather; heat
< cold, air, damp	> cold applications
< wind, **coffee**, alcohol	**> being carried**

Cimicifuga (3)

Labor-like pains, sharp pains dart side to side, back pain to sciatica, restless; **pain across pelvis from hip to hip** (Bell); profuse, dark, **coagulated** blood; pain in ovarian region shoots upward and down anterior surface of thighs; menses always irregular; offensive with backache, nervousness; after pains with great sensitiveness and **intolerance to pain**; facial blemishes in young women; greater flow = greater pain; sore and tender along track of pain; thirsty; chilly.

< menses, suppressed emotions	> warm wraps; eating
< alcohol; night	> open air; pressure

< air, damp, cold, wind, night
< change of weather
< hot and cold; sitting
< AM

> continued motion
> grasping things

Colocynthis (2)

Better pressure at first then heat; **bends over double** (Opium); **> bending double**; sharp stabbing pain, intermittent, left side; **boring pain in ovary**; **restlessness**; wants abdomen supported by pressure; bearing down pains; **waves of violent cutting**; **gripping**; **grasping pains**; vomits from pain; anger, easily vexed; thirsty.

< emotions, anger; **vexation**
< lying on painless side
< night, in bed, drafts
< taking cold
< least food

> hard pressure, coffee
> heat, rest, gentle motion
> after stool, passing gas
> lying with head bent forward

Dioscorea (2)

Severe cramps, **> bending backward**; **cramps in fingers and toes alternate with abdominal cramps**; pain radiates from uterus; vivid dreams; **unbearable sharp**, **cutting**, **twisting**, **griping or grinding pains**; pain darts, radiates to distant parts, in paroxysms; suddenly cease then start.

< doubling up, **lying**
< evening, night

> stretching out; open air
> motion; bending backwards
> hard pressure
> standing erect

Kali carb (3)

Left hypochondrial pain;left abdomen, menses early (Calc), profuse or **too late**, **pale and scanty** with soreness of genitals; back pains pass down through gluteal muscles with cutting abdominal pains; pains from abdomen to chest, through left labium; delayed menses in young girls with chest symptoms; **complaints after parturition**; uterine bleeding of constant oozing after copious flow with violent backache > with sitting and pressure; colic then irritating menses; thirst, **chilly**.

< cold, air, water, draft, after cold
< 2–3 AM
< winter; before menses
< on painful or left side
< loss of fluids, post labor
< after coition
< soup and coffee

> warmth, warm moist
> sitting with elbows on knees
> open air; **bending double**
> during the day

Pulsatilla (2)

Sadness and/or weeping before menses, nausea, chilliness, gastrointestinal complaints; **sensation of band around throat just before menses**, changeable flow month to month; suppressed menses from wet feet; too late scanty, thick, dark **clotted**, **intermittent**, **changeable** menses; downward pressure, painful flow intermits; back pain, diarrhea during or after menses; must bend double; **thirstless**, anemic, stuffy rooms aggravate.

< warmth, of room, air, bed
< wet feet; **suppressions**
< rest; **beginning motion**,
< eating rich foods; **fats**, eggs
< lying; **evenings**
< lying on left or painless side

> cold; **fresh air**
> uncovering
> erect posture
> gentle motion
> consolation,. after crying

Consider:

Graphites (2)

Marked constipation with dysmenorrhea; low back pain with nausea and vomiting; menses **too late**; pale; scanty flow with tearing epigastric pain and itching **before**; coryza, cough, morning sickness during menses; aversion to coitus; **excoriations**, **cracks or fissures**, scanty, foul, thin, sticky, corrosive secretions; gushes of pale, thin **profuse white** excoriating **leukorrhea rather than menses**; voice lacks control, **chilly**.

< cold, drafts
< menses; light
< empty swallowing
< fats, hot drinks

> open air; eating; touch

< warmth of bed; night
< scratching; wet feet

Magnesia phos

Cell salt, pain > with heat and pressure; **membranous dysmenorrhea**; early menses swelling of external parts; ovarian neuralgia, menses dark, stringy; vaginismus, **sudden** paroxysms of pain; tarry menses leaving a fast stain, flowing at night, **chilly**.

< cold, **air**, uncovering, water	**> warmth**, **hot bath**
< lying on right side	> pressure; rubbing
< touch, night, periodicity	> doubling up; friction
< milk; exhaustion	

Ustilago

Burning pains, swelling of ovaries, especially left; menses excessive, flows easily, gushing, intermittent or continuous bleeding of bright red or **dark blood**; coagulated, clotted blood, may form in long strings; **cervix is spongy**, **friable** and **bleeds easily**; bleeding is < touch; vicarious menses from lungs or rectum; metrorrhagia, **passive**, **constant flow**, after abortion, with fibroid tumors; soreness of uterus and ovaries, left ovarian pain which extends to the uterus; uterine pains > with flow (Lach); pains shoot down thighs, to hips, into groin, especially the left; bearing down sensation (Lil t, Sep); **uterine fibroids**; ***hair and nail loss***.

< touch; motion	> flow (uterine pains)
< menses	
< pressure (ovaries)	

Symptoms in Kent's Repertory	**Page**
Mind, Irritability, menses	59
Mind, Sadness, menses during	77
Head, Pain, menses before/during	142
Stomach, Nausea, menses during	508
Rectum, Constipation, menses during	608
Genitalia-F, leukorrhea, menses between	722
Genitalia-F, Menses, painful, dysmenorrhea	727

EYE INJURIES, INFLAMMATION

There are many types of conditions which affect the eye both internally and externally. **Vision loss** from infection affects millions of people worldwide and is more prevalent in areas with poor nutrition and sanitation. Vision loss from **glaucoma**, **diabetes** and **trauma** is more commonly seen in the industrialized nations.

It is important that the practitioner be aware of the type of condition being treated and its possible outcomes before prescribing. While homeopathic medicine has proven to be highly effective in the treatment of **diseases of the eye**, the opinion of an expert in the field of optometry or ophthalmology should be obtained when you are uncertain of what is occurring.

Aconite (3)

Sensation of **heat**, **dryness in eye**; eye is red, inflamed; **lids red**, **hard**, **swollen**; profuse tearing following exposure to dry, cold wind, from **snow blindness**; sensation as if there is sand in the eye, foreign body; good for **pain of scratched cornea following foreign body extraction**; < light.

< night; **warm room** — > open air
< light
< cold winds

Arnica (3)

Retinal hemorrhage, from **trauma**; **eyes feel sore**, **bruised** and weary, especially after prolonged use; dizziness with closing eyes; double vision from trauma; **bloodshot** (Nat m); tall objects appear to lean foreword; burning pains with flowing, excoriating tears; swelling of lids with ecchymosis; contraction of pupils; fixed, anxious look.

< injuries, **jarring**, touch — **> lying**

< over exertion
< damp cold

Euphrasia (2)

Acrid lacrimation which is **profuse**, **eyes water constantly** and feel hot, may be accompanied by a bland nasal discharge; discharge from eyes is sticky, thick and excoriating, must blink often in order to clear eye; feeling of pressure in eye; catarrhal conjunctivitis, with redness of the eye; small blisters on cornea; tearing < in open air, **lying** or with coughing; eye pains alternate with abdominal pains; cataracts; lancinating pains and photophobia in the bright light; dryness and pressure in the eyes; ptosis (Caust, Gels, Led).

< sunlight; **warmth**	**> open air**
< wind, evenings	> wiping eyes; in the dark

Hamamelis

For the effects of trauma with a **bruised**, **soreness** sensation (Arn); when the vessels are very injected; eyes are bloodshot; capillary hemorrhages, dark, fluid like and may cause or relieve weakness; will expedite resorption of intraocular hemorrhage; painful weakness of the eyes; ***sensation as if eyes are being forced out of sockets which is > with pressure***, **< a few moments afterward**; soreness after operation.

< pressure on eyes (after a brief initial amelioration)
< warm, moist open air
< jarring, motion

Ledum (2)

Puncture wounds, contusions, especially with a **feeling of coldness** in the eye; aching pains; extravasation of blood in lids, conjunctiva or in the eye; **bloodshot eyes** (Arn, Ham), **bruising**; acrid tearing which excoriates lids and cheeks; hemorrhage after surgery; ptosis of the lid (Caust, Euph, Gels); suppuration of eyes with discharge of pus; inflammation with agglutination, tearing pains; vision difficult with sparks before eyes; itching of eyes, internal canthi.

< heat, **warmth**	**> cold**
< motion	> lying down

Mercurius cor

Iritis, acute flare-ups with a rapid onset; excessive photophobia, with **acrid and profuse lachrymation**; **severe tearing**, **lancinating pains**; **eyes very sore**, after attack; pain behind eyeballs, with a sensation that they are being forced outward; **iris appears irregular in shape**, **muddy in color**, **thick**, **with little contraction or dilation**; burning pain with dryness; hemorrhagic iritis; ulcerations on the cornea which are deep (opp. Sulph); double vision; small vesicles or blisters on the cornea; night blindness; pains come on due to fatigue, bright lights shining in eyes at night; < extremes of temperatures; **thirsty**, with a moist mouth.

< night	> rest
< extremes of cold, heat	

Natrum mur

Weakness, **stiffness of ocular muscles**; weakness from reading, overuse (Ruta); letters run together; **weakness of vision** related to **weakness of internal rectus muscles** (opp. Cupr acet, Gels; Phos); **painful with looking downward**; burning and acrid lachrymation; bruised feeling with headaches, especially in children; stricture and suppuration of the lachrymal duct (Fl-ac, Puls, Rhus t, Sil); **difficulty seeing with artificial light**; fiery, zigzag appearance around objects.

< mental exertion	> open air
< heat	
< over use	

Phosphorus

Atrophy of the optic nerve; paresis of the ocular muscles (Caust, Gels, Nat m, Nux v, Rhus t); glaucoma (Osmium); **degenerative changes**, in the elderly, with soreness and difficulty with bright lights and changes in objects being seen; **thrombosis of retinal vessels**; sensation as if a veil or mist were covering eyes; **green halo around the light or candle** (Osmium), **letters may appear red**; diplopia; partial loss of vision from use of tobacco (Nux v); fatigue of eyes, which may be better with shading eyes; pain in orbital bones; edema of lids and around eyes; **thirsty**; chilly.

< touch
< weather changes

> in the dark

Pulsatilla

Complete loss of vision, with no apparent cause, **especially during menses**; dimness of vision with a sensation as if something was covering the eyes (Phos), causing person to to rub them, < wind; **profuse**, **thick**, **bland yellowish discharge**; optic nerve paralysis; itching and burning of the eyes, < evenings; **inflammation of the lids with agglutination**; conjunctivitis; ophthalmia neonatorum, especially gonorrheal; dryness of the eyes, especially during sleep; profuse lachrymation, < wind; eyes very sensitive to light causing sharp pains; diffusion of light and luminous circles with viewing bright objects; funduscopic exam shows enlarged vessels; thirstless, weepy, chilly.

< heat, **evenings**
< before menses

> open air
> cold applications
> gentle motion

Ruta

Good remedy for **eyestrain following close-up work or reading small print, especially if followed by a headache** (Arg n, Nat m); **difficulty with accommodation**; **paralysis of the ciliary muscles**; sensation of a deep pressure in the orbits, of pressure over the eyebrow; eyes feel hot, painful, strained; **dimness of vision** (Puls); ***spasm of lower lid with lachrymation when it stops;*** bruised feeling of the eye; retinal detachments (Naph); red or green halo around lights; lachrymation from itching of inner canthus and in open air; weakness of vision with pain and headaches.

< cold, wet weather
< over exertion
< damp, wind

> warmth
> rubbing, scratching

Staphysagria (2)

Sensation of warmth, heat in the eye (Euph, Sulph); ***eyes feel dry,* with lachrymation**; sunken eyes with blue, raised rings around them; pupils dilated; burning sensation in eyes when writing, when looking at the sun, causing profuse, hot tearing which excoriates the cheeks; iritis (Merc c) with bursting, burning pains in eyeball, temple and side of the face, < evenings to mornings (follows Aconite); agglutination of eyes in AM; spasmodic closing of lids; sensation as if a hard substance is under the lid causing pain (see styes); sparks before eyes, in the dark; black flashes before eyes; good remedy for **pain from healing lacerations** of the globe or cornea; very sensitive; chilly.

< anger — > warmth, rest
< loss of fluids
< touch

Sulphur (2)

Painful inflammation from foreign bodies, vessels are dilated, bright to dark red; trembling of eyes and eyelids; objects seem more distant than they really are; photophobia; **halo around lights** (Osm, Phos, Puls); **burning pains**, especially with ulceration of the lid margins; good in chronic ophthalmia when there is intense burning and itching; first stages of corneal ulceration; interstitial keratitis; cornea has a ground glass like appearance; pain which extends into the head, < movement of the eyes; unequal pupils; eyes feel hot (Euph, Staph); agglutination of lids; eyes very sensitive to light (Nat m); objects appear to be yellow; Consider Sulphuric acid if intraocular hemorrhage is due to trauma; thirsty; chilly but can be < heat.

< becoming heated — > open air

Symphytum (3)

Excellent remedy for **eye pain after a blow**, **from trauma**; ***orbital fractures;*** eyelids closed due to spasm; often there is no visible injury to the eye; sensation as if the eyelid has passed over a bulb on the eye, with closing; desire to rest eyes.

< touch, blows
< injuries

Consider:

Bothrops

Blindness due to retinal hemorrhage or thrombosis; hemorrhages of the conjunctiva; day time blindness; hemiplegia with inability to speak, articulate.

Kalmia latifolia

Eye pains with retinitis, chorioretinitis, **sclero-iritis**, ocular paresis; ptosis; impairment of vision; **stiff, drawing sensation in the eye with movement**; < leaning forward, looking down.

Naphthaline

Retinal detachment, with shiny bodies in the vitreous humor; patchy deposits and infiltration of the retina; exudation of retina, choroid and ciliary body; amblyopia; cataracts (Phos) and **corneal opacity** or a white patchy material on retina, which increases in size; eyes are painful, bloodshot (Nat m), inflamed; patient may have a staggering gait, sudden onset of symptoms, generalized muscular twitchings.

Osmium

Remedy for glaucoma (Phos), especially if vision is iridescent; violent pains which are above and below the orbit; patient reports seeing a **green halo around the light or candle**; increase of intraocular pressure; dimness of sight and photophobia.

Pilocarpus

Generalized eye strain; irritability of ciliary muscles; fatigue of the eye from the slightest use; heat, burning in the eyes; **smarting eye pains**; spasm of accommodation, when distant objects appear hazy, blurry, then vision returns and becomes blurry again; **pupils do not accommodate to light** (Merc c); retinal images remain long after viewing the object; **near sightedness**; twitching of lids; white spots before eyes; exophthalmos; opacities in vitreous body; nervous, tremulous individuals who get headaches with vertigo and nausea with using eyes; **Contraindicated in heart failure patients in low doses**.

< cold; exhaustion

Rhus tox

Orbital cellulitis and pustular inflammations; red, swollen and edematous; profuse yellow pus (Puls); **iritis following cold and damp exposure**; eye pain < with turning, or pressing on eye; old injuries to eyes; profuse gushing of hot tears with opening of lids; ulceration of the cornea (Merc c, Sulph); **aggravated in cold, wet weather**; **conjunctivitis**.

Symptoms in Kent's Repertory	**Page**
Eye, Bleeding from	235
Eye, Close, spasmodic closure	236
Eye, Ecchymosis	238
Eye, Inflammation, foreign bodies/injuries after	242
Eye, Injected	244
Eye, Pain, from a blow	249
Eye, Pain, sore, bruised, tender	258
Eye, Swollen	267
Vision, Blurred	271
Vision, Loss of Vision, injuries to eye	282

FLATULENCE

Gas or **"passing wind"** is often a result of incomplete digestion. Gut bacteria act upon incompletely digested foods such as carbohydrates, fats and proteins, releasing by-products of their digestion such as methane or other gasses. This condition may occur periodically and follow eating certain foods such as beans, milk or wheat and is associated with poor enzyme production. If excessive gas production occurs frequently, then you must consider that the person has a serious digestive and absorption problem that needs attention.

If a correlation can be made with the type of food that is causing the flatulence, then its elimination is in order to correct the problem. Flatulence associated with diarrhea may signal a pathologic process which must be evaluated by a physician.

Argentum nit (3)

Distension of entire abdomen and body, severe loud eructation and flatulence; fear; stage fright; very nervous that brings on condition; colic, stitching pain on left side: **fluids go right through him**.

< emotion; **anxiety**	> cool, open air, bath
< in room; sugar; drinking	> hard pressure; motion
< lying right side; looking down	> eructations
< crowds: warmth	
< sweets; after eating	
< left side	

Carbo veg (3)

Similar to Lycopodium and China but more diarrhea; bubble of hot metal that goes to extremities and head; paralytic ileus with gas over entire abdomen; **flatulent colic** > passing gas; flatus hot, moist, offensive; tense from flatulence; **eructations** from undigested food; **air hunger**, gas < upper abdomen, thirst, chilly.

< warmth, **depletion**
< exhausting diseases; old age
< high living, rich food
< walking in open air
< pressure of clothes
< cooling off
< cold night air, extreme temperatures

> eructations
> cool air; fanning
> elevating feet

China (3)

Flatulence and eructations; distension of entire abdomen; belching of bitter fluid **gives no relief** (Mag p); stool with much flatulence, weakening ; flatulent colic > bending double (Mag p); **thirst and thirstless**, chilly.

< touch, **vital losses**
< jarring, noise
< alternate days
< cold, draft, wind
< open air
< fruit, milk

> hard pressure
> loose clothes

Colchicum (3)

After eating fruit gets gas and cannot let go of it; distension of abdomen with gas; **smell of food causes nausea even to fainting**; borborygmus; cecum and ascending colon much distended;**cold and weak but sensitive and restless**; **acute smell**; **thirstless and thirst**.

< motion; touch, night
< sundown to sunrise
< weather– cold, damp, changing
< stretching
< slight exertion

> **doubling up**
> sitting; warmth; rest

Lycopodium (3)

Abdomen distended like a drum; sounds hollow; lower abdomen, offensive flatulence; sour burping occurs immediately after eating; constant sense of fermentation in abdomen; rolling of flatulence; dyspepsia due to farinaceous and fermentable foods; **much noisy flatulence** < lower bowels; thirstless, chilly.

< pressure of clothes
< warmth; awaking, wind
< eating, to satiety, oysters
< 4–8 PM, indigestion
< right side

> warm drinks; food
> cold applications
> motion, eructations, urinating

Magnesia phos

Flatulent colic forces patient to bend double (Coloc); **relieved by rubbing, warmth, pressure**; **belches gas which does not relieve** (China); **bloated**; **full sensation in abdomen**; **loosens clothes, walks about and constantly passes flatus**.

< lying on right side
< cold; touch; night
< milk
< exhaustion

> warmth
> bending double
> pressure; friction

Plumbum met (3)

Intense gas; intense constipation like something is pushing in abdomen; **colic radiates to all parts of the body**; **abdominal wall feels drawn by a string to spine**; obstructed flatus with intense colic; foul eructations; thirst; chilly.

< clear weather; open air
< exertion; motion; company
< grasping smooth objects
< touch; night

> hard pressure
> rubbing
> physical exertion

Raphanus (2)

Paralytic ileus with gas at splenic flexure; great accumulation and incarceration of flatus; **no flatus emitted upward or downward**; griping around navel; **post-operative gas pains**; vomits fecal matter; thirsty.

Symptoms in Kent's Repertory

	Page
Rectum, Flatus, diarrhea during	617
Rectum, Flatus, loud/sputtering	618
Rectum, Flatus, urging for stool, only flatus passed	618
Rectum, Fullness	618

GALLSTONES—GALLBLADDER PAIN

An "attack" of **gallstones** often shows itself as right upper quadrant pain soon after a meal, especially one that is high in fats. The patient will often be doubled over with severe pain and have difficulty breathing. **Gallbladder disease** is not a disease of the gallbladder but rather one of the liver. The gallbladder is simply a storage vesicle for the bile which is produced by the liver.

Another condition which may be similar to a gallstone attack is **cholecystitis**. Cholecystitis is due to an inflammation of the gallbladder and can often have similar symptoms, but will have a higher temperature associated with it. While a gallstone attack is not life-threatening, the pain associated with it may be severe enough to cause the patient to go into shock. Cholecystitis can lead to sepsis and shock as well and needs to be evaluated by a physician.

Berberis (3)

Colic, followed by jaundice; shooting, burning pressure in region of gallbladder; spasmodic pains confined to a small spot; stitching pains; worse pressure, extending to gallbladder; stitching pains in front of kidneys extending to liver, spleen, stomach, groin; slimy dark urine with heavy sediment; radiating pains from one point; mentally and physically tired; **breathing arrested from pain**; shooting and tearing pain in region of right hypochondrium spreading inward to epigastrium, across to the left or down to the umbilicus; excellent remedy for renal colic due to stones; thirsty.

< motion, **jarring**, stepping hard
< rising from sitting   > fatigue; urinating

Calcarea carb (2)

Great chilliness during attack; pain darts from right to left with profuse sweat, abdominal spasms, colic; cutting colic in epigastrium, has to bend double, clench hands, writhes in agony; incarcerated flatus; **gallstone colic**; cannot bear tight clothing around abdomen (Nux v); sour discharges; thirst for cold water at night; **thirsty**, chilly.

< **cold**, **air**, wet, **bathing**	> dry climate, weather
< cooling off; change of weather	> lying on painful side
< exertion, mental, physical, ascending	
< pressure of clothes; anxiety	
< milk; awaking	
< full moon	

Carduus marianus (3)

Region sensitive to pressure; crawling sensation like passage of a small body through a narrow canal, on posterior side of liver from right to left and to pit of stomach. Left lobe of liver very sensitive; fullness, soreness with moist skin; stools bright yellow, **hard**, **difficult**, **knotty**; alternates with diarrhea; swelling of gallbladder; vomits acrid bile or blood; golden yellow urine; difficulty rising.

< lying on left side; beer	> belching
< eating; touch; motion	
< cellars	
< from stooping	

Chelidonium (2)

Chill with intense pain in region of gallbladder, quickly extending down and across navel into intestines; vomiting and clay colored stools; **pain in liver shooting to under right scapula**; enlarged liver, distention; stool hard, round balls like sheep dung; bright yellow, pasty, float; **alternating diarrhea and constipation**; prefers hot food and drink; thirsty; chilly.

< motion; cough; touch	> hot food; eating
< change of weather	> milk; pressure
< 4 AM; 4 PM	> hot bath; bending backward
< right side	

Chenopodium (2)

Severe pain in region of lower inner angle of right scapula to chest; cold feet up to knees; tired legs and knees; constipation; stool like sheep dung, hard and knotty.

China (3)

Obstruction of gallbladder with colic; periodic recurrence, yellow skin and sclera; constipation with dark greenish scybala; sensitive to least pressure; much flatulent colic; > bending double (Coloc); **tympanic abdomen**; pain right hypochondrium; internal coldness of stomach and abdomen; stools undigested, yellow; frothy, **painless**; **profuse**, **exhausting discharges**; **gallstone colic**; loud belching with no relief; **drenching sweats at night**; **thirsty**; chilly.

< vital fluid loss; **touch**	> hard pressure
< jarring, noise	> loose clothes
< alternates days, **periodically**	> bending double
< cold, drafts, wind, open air	> open air; warmth
< eating; fruit; milk	
< mental exertion	

Dioscorea (2)

Cutting pains, change locations; sudden shifting of pains to different parts, **appear in remote locales as fingers**, **toes**; rumbling with passing of much flatus; griping, cutting in hypogastric region, with intermittent cutting pain in stomach, intestines; **sharp pains from liver shooting upward to right nipple**; **unbearable sharp**, **cutting**, **twisting**, **grinding pains**.

< doubling up; lying	> stretching out or bending backwards
< at menses	> motion; open air
< tea; eating;	> hard pressure
< evening and night	

Lycopodium (3)

Immediate bloating after a meal; constant sense of fermentation in abdomen; upper left side; sensitive liver; pain shoots across lower abdomen from right to left; brown spots on abdomen; stool **hard**, **difficult**, **small**, incomplete; **much noisy flatulence**; **awakes angry**; chilly.

< pressure of clothes; **warmth**	**> warm drinks**; food
< awaking; wind	> cold applications
< eating to satiety, oysters	> motion; eructations

< indigestion; 4–8 PM
< right to left, from above downward

> urinating
> after midnight
> being uncovered

Natrum sulph (3)

Icterus, vomiting of bile; liver sore to touch with sharp pains; cannot bear tight clothing around waist; < lying on left side; **flatus** especially in ascending colon < before breakfast; diarrhea yellow, watery stool; **loose AM stools**; involuntary stool with flatus; **rumbling**, **gurgling in bowels then sudden gushing**, **noisy**, **spluttering stool**; chilly; piercing pains at left ribs to left hip.

< damp, weather, night air, cellars
< lying on left side; pressure
< head injuries; lifting; touch
< late evening; wind, light
< music

> open air
> change of position

Consider:

Baptisia (2)

Right side affected mainly; distended and rumbling; soreness over region of gallbladder with diarrhea; **stools offensive**, **dark**, **bloody**; thirsty.

Belladonna (3)

Distended, hot; protrusion of transverse colon; tender, swollen abdomen; cutting pains across abdomen; stitches on left side; extreme sensitiveness to touch (Lach); thirsty, thirstless.

Chionanthus (2)

Colic, sensation like a string tied around intestines in umbilical region, every now and then is drawn tight then gradually loosened; somewhat > by lying on stomach, abdomen; **enlarged liver with jaundice**; stools are clay colored, soft, yellow and pasty.

Nux vomica (2)

Jaundice, aversion to food; fainting; gallstones; constipation; cannot bear tight clothes on abdomen, **bruised soreness of abdom-**

inal walls (Apis, Sulph); colic from uncovering; flatulent distension with colic; thirsty; chilly.

Podophyllum (1)

Jaundice with gallstones; pain from stomach to gallbladder with excessive nausea; **constantly rubbing and stroking hypochondrium**; alternating constipation and diarrhea; **sensation of weakness or sinking**; distension; heat and emptiness, thirsty.

Taraxacum

Enlargement of liver; sharp stitching pains in left side; rumbling sensation in abdomen; chilliness after eating; weakness after eating; bitter taste in mouth; profuse night sweats.

Symptoms in Kent's Repertory	**Page**
Abdomen, Clothing, sensitive to	541
Abdomen, Distention, painful	545
Abdomen, Distention, tympanic	545
Abdomen, Pain, hypochondria, extending to back	563
Abdomen, Pain, hypochondria, walking, extending to back	564
Abdomen, Pain, liver, colic gallstones	568
Abdomen, Pain, liver, extending to back	569
Generalities, Food, fat agg.	1362

See **Abdominal Inflammation**.

GASTRIC—
DUODENAL ULCERS

Gastric ulceration will present with a wide variety of symptoms which range from a mild, constant nausea to a severe doubling-over with pain and shock from perforation. Usually the person knows what the problem is, as they have had previous attacks or symptoms. Attacks are often caused by stress, ingestion of acid foods or fluids, and are alleviated by antacids.

Bleeding can occur and may range from a mild to severe blood loss, resulting in nausea and vomiting and blackened stools. A considerable amount of blood can be lost with mildly blackened or tarry stools if the condition continues for more than five days. An increase in the person's pulse rate as well as pale mucous membranes of the mouth and nail beds should alert you to blood loss. Additionally, a **perforated ulcer** will cause **peritonitis** (infection of the abdominal cavity) which, along with the blood loss, is potentially life-threatening.

Argentum nit (3)

Specific for ileus; burning, gripping pain, much distension; **cannot belch, which is very loud if able to do so, also flatus, gives some relief**; black vomitus; nausea, retching, vomiting of glaring mucus; painful spot over stomach that **radiates to all parts of abdomen**; gnawing pain, burning, constriction; **great desire for sweets**; ulcerative pain on left side under ribs; desires cheese and salt; **belching** with most gastric ailments; **violent pains like splinters**; nervous, impulsive, hurried; timid; anxious; astringent; sour, bitter taste of vomitus; **thirsty**, chilly.

< emotions, **anxiety**, suspense	**> cool**, **air**, bath
< in room; sugar; shut in places	> hard pressure; motion
< lying on right side; looking down	> eructations
< drinking; crowds	
< warmth in any form; night	

< cold food; after eating
< left side

Arsenicum alb (3)

Irritates, destruction of mucous membranes; **intense burning pains** by pylorus; nausea and vomiting of coffee ground substance (Phos); black tarry stools; **cannot bear the sight or smell of food** (Colch); **great thirst**; **drinks much but in sips**; nausea and vomiting after eating, drinking; **anxiety** in pit of stomach; craves acids, coffee; irritable stomach; seems raw; terrible pain and dyspnea with gastralgia; great exhaustion, coldness; craves milk; **ill effects of vegetable diet**, **watery fruits**; everything seems to lodge in esophagus, seems nothing will pass; **restlessness**; **fears**; chilly.

< cold, **ices**, **drinks**, **foods**, air	**> hot**, **applications**, **food**
< periodically, **after midnight 2 AM**	> hot drinks; wraps
< vegetables; **drinking**	> motion
< exertion; tobacco; lying on part	**> elevating head**
< eruptions; suppressed; undeveloped	> sitting erect, company
< seashore; wet weather; right side	> sweating

Bismuth (3)

Water is vomited as soon as it reaches stomach (Ars); eructations after drinking; **burning**, **feeling of a load**; eats for several days until vomits; slow digestion with **fetid** eructations; pain from stomach to spine; gastritis; **better cold drinks** but vomits with a full stomach; inexpressible pain in stomach; pressure from a load in one spot alternates with burning, cramping pain; **desire for company**; **anguish**; discontented; craves cold drinks; white coated tongue; sweet metallic taste.

< eating, overeating	> cold, drinks, applications
	> bending backward; motion

Chelidonium (3)

Pain radiates to inferior border of right scapula; intensely hot drinks makes things better; **eating relieves temporarily**; bad odor from mouth; **drowsy**; thirsty; chilly.

< motion; cough; touch
< weather changes
< 4 AM, 4 PM

> hot food; eating
> milk; pressure; hot bath
> bending backward

Hydrastis (2)

Mucus everywhere, feels like a hernia at pylorus(hiatal); empty feeling but no appetite; fullness after eating; yellow mucus; sore feeling in stomach is constant; **bitter taste**; pain as if from a hard-cornered substance; epigastric pulsation; cannot eat bread or vegetables; gastritis, ulcers and cancer of stomach; constipation; ropey mucus; cutting pain from liver to right scapula, < lying on right side or back.

< air, inhaling cold, dry wind, open
< slight bleeding, old age; washing

Kali bic (2)

Most common remedy, deep penetrating ulcers; intense pain left of xyphoid very localized, sometimes goes to back vertebrae; after alcohol (beer, whiskey); after eating, food sits like weight in stomach right away; desires beer and acids; **round ulcers of stomach**; alcohol abuse, dipsomania, belching sour after meals; nausea after eating; may vomit, bright yellow water, tastes sour; gastric symptoms > eating; cannot digest meat, milk; gastritis, nausea and vomiting after beer; cutting abdominal pains soon after eating; headache, constipation, poor sleep; **adhesive secretions**, **thick**, **sticky**, **stringy**, **tough**; pains in small spots, wander, finally to stomach; pain comes with loss of appetite and **thirst for beer** or acids which can aggravate; thirsty, **chilly**.

< cold, damp, open air, undressing
< AM; 2–3 AM, after sleep
< hot weather; **alcohol**, **beer**
< suppressed catarrh

> heat; motion

Lycopodium (3)

Bloating after eating; sensitive to clothing around abdomen (Lach, Nux v, Puls); dyspepsia from farinaceous and fermentable food, beans; excessive hunger; awakes at night with hunger; **incom-**

plete burning eructations rise only to pharynx, burns for hours; eating little creates fullness; food tastes sour; desires sweets; sinking sensation, < night; **awakes angry**; gnawing in stomach; **noisy flatus, gas low down moves down**; pains > walking slowly, lying, < sitting; weakness of digestion.

< pressure of clothes	**> warm drinks**, food
< warmth; awaking, wind	> cold applications; uncovered
< eating to satiety; oysters	> motion; eructations
< indigestion; 4–8 PM	> urinating; after midnight
< right side; right to left; above to below	

Nux vomica (3)

Nausea in AM after eating; weight and pain in stomach; worse eating and for some time after; nausea and vomiting with retching; ravenous hunger especially before an attack of dyspepsia; **region of stomach very sensitive to pressure** (Ars, Bry, Lach); pressure and bloating **several hours after eating**; desires stimulants, fats; wants to vomit but cannot, belch but cannot; dyspepsia $\frac{1}{2}$–1 hour after eating (Puls), pain right after eating; similar to Kali bich; **angry**, **impatient**, **ugly**; bruised soreness of abdomen (Apis); sensitive, critical; food lies like a heavy knot in stomach; gastric pains into back, chest; > vomiting; **easily chilled**; thirsty.

< early AM; **cold**, **air, drafts**	**> free discharges**; naps
< mental exertion, disturbed sleep	> wrapping head; resting
< high living; **coffee**, liquor, drugs	> hot drinks; milk; moist air
< sedentary habits, overeating	> evenings
< slightest causes, anger, noise,odors	> strong pressure, touch

Phosphorus (3)

Pain around pylorus, about to perforate; pain goes away 5–10 minutes after cold drink; develops fullness, pain after eating; emesis looks like coffee grounds (Ars) with bright red blood, **postoperative vomiting; vomits water as soon as it gets warm in stomach**

(Ars & Bismuth vomits it immediately); burning pain > with cold; empty weakness 11 AM; gnawing hunger; always eating, cold things; sour taste and eructations after meals; hunger soon after meals; region of stomach painful to touch or on walking; **ill effects of eating too much salt**; waterbrash; craves salt; **thirsty**, chilly.

< lying on left; painful side,
< lying on back
< slight emotions; talking
< touch ;odors; light
< cold hands(in water); open air
< warm ingesta; **salt**
< weather, changes, windy, cold
< thunderstorms
< AM & PM
< mental exertion

> eating; sleep; cold food
> sleep
> cold water to face
> rubbing
> sitting up; in dark
> lying on right side

Pulsatilla (3)

Pain, colic, gripping $\frac{1}{2}$–1 hour after eating (Nux v); food sits like a lump, eats too much; sourness; heartburn; **waterbrash**; cramps in stomach with water rising to throat and expelled; **taste of food remains for a long time**; **averse to fats**, **warm food and drink**; **bitter taste**; pain as if from a subcutaneous ulcer; dyspepsia with great tightness after a meal, must loosen clothes (Lach, Lyc, Nux v); **weight** as from a stone, especially in AM, awakening; gnawing hungry feeling (Abies c); **thirstless**, **mild**, **weepy**; **changing shifting symptoms**; abdominal pains to the groin; craves acids which disagree; desires cold, bubbly drinks; **desires fresh air**.

< warmth, **air**, **room**, bed
< getting feet wet
< suppressions, **evenings**
< beginning motion; **lying**
< fats; **rich foods**; **eating**
< eating ices, **rest**

> cold, **fresh open air**
> uncovering
> erect posture
> gentle motion; weeping
> cold food and drink

Consider:

Bryonia (3)

Nausea, faintness when rising up; abnormal hunger, loss of taste; vomiting of bile and water immediately after eating; **stomach sensitive to touch** (Ars, Nux v); **pressure like a stone in stomach after eating**; **thirst for large quantities of cold water**; **averse to motion**; **thirsty**.

Carduus mar (3)

Nausea; **retching**; **vomiting of green**, **acid fluid**; stitches left side of stomach; bitter taste, averse to salt, meat.

Chamomilla (2)

Foul eructations; nausea after coffee; sweats after eating, drinking; averse to warm drinks; pressive gastralgia as if from a stone; **irritable**, consider for acute pain; **thirsty**.

China (3)

Tender, cold abdomen; vomits undigested food; distended; hungry with no appetite; averse to milk; **flatulence**, **belching** of undigested **food gives no relief**; darting pains across hypogastric region, chilly, **thirsty**.

Cuprum met (3)

Violent spasms, pains in stomach and abdomen; vomiting; violent tenesmus; **cramps, spasms of all kinds**; **tense abdomen**, **colic > pressure and bending double**; **> cold drinks**; **thirsty**.

Graphites (3)

Drinks much hot milk, hot fluids, food; **intense pain > with eating**; mainly for gastritis; **hot drinks disagree**; stomach > hot drinks; burning in stomach causes **hunger**; **constrictive pain in stomach**; nausea and vomiting after each meal; averse to heat; nauseated by sweets; **chilly**.

Kreosotum (2)

Vomits hours after eating, looks as if they have first eaten; soreness > eating; painful hard spot, hematemesis; nausea, icy cold epigastrium; stomach aggravated by eating smoked meats, fish; sensation of a painful lump or ball in the epigastrium, tight feeling in stomach which causes patient to loosen clothing; good for cancer of the stomach; chilly.

Stannum (3)

Smell of cooking causes vomiting; pain better pressure but sore to touch; **empty feeling in stomach**; **colic relieved by pressure**, **pains increase gradually then slowly subside**; chilly.

Gastric—Duodenal Ulcers: See under **Abdominal Inflammation**

HAYFEVER—ALLERGIES

Allergies and **hayfever** can affect most people at some time in their life and are often regarded as more of a nuisance than an indication that there is something wrong with the immune system. Most often encountered in the spring due to wind-borne pollens, this condition affects the nose, mouth, eyes and throat, head and mental state. Causes will vary from person to person and may be due to changes in seasons, genetic predisposition, amount of exposure to allergens, and levels of stress.

There may be a gradual or abrupt onset of tearing, itching of the nose and mouth, headache, sneezing and nasal discharge, and eventual obstruction. The person may have swollen, puffy and red eyes, difficulty with hearing, and there may be wheezing with taking a breath. Symptoms may range from mild to severe.

Allium cepa (3)

Nose and eyes stream; severe sneezing with increased frequency; sneezing especially with entering a warm room; **copious watery extremely acrid discharge**; sensation of a lump at root of nose; coryza with headache, cough, hoarseness; eyes red with **burning**, smarting lachrymation, **sensitive to light**; bland lachrymation better in open air; burning of eyelids, lips and nostrils sore; thirsty.

< indoors; evenings
< warm room
< in AM; from flowers

> open air; cold room

Arsenicum alb (2)

Thin, **water**, **excoriating discharge**; violent tickle on inside of nose; dull throbbing headache; sneezing **without** relief; nose feels **stopped up**; **burning**, bleeding of nose; **burning of eyes with acrid lacrimation**; lids red, ulcerated, scabby, granulated; **intense photophobia**; painful inflammation of eyes; **restlessness**; sneezing with biting watery coryza; sensitive to smells, odor of food; sight or thinking of food; **burning thirst for cold drinks**, **drinks in sips**; **chilly**.

< cold, **drinks**, air, food
< every 14 days
< after midnight, 2 AM,
< vegetables, **drinking**
< eruptions; **exertion**
< lying on affected part
< tobacco; right side
< wet weather; seashore
< weather changes

> hot, **applications**, food drink
> wrapped up; motion
> head elevated
> sitting erect; company
> sweating

Arsenicum iod (2)

Thin, **watery**, **irritating**; **excoriating discharge from anterior**, **posterior nares**; **sneezing**; irritation in nose with constant desire to sneeze, nose swollen; **chronic catarrh**, profuse, thick, yellow; ulcers of nose; nasal mucosa **sore**, **excoriated**; aggravated by sneezing; nose drips water; aching malar bones; burning in nose and throat; discharge is thin acutely; thick chronically; thirsty, chilly.

< dry, cold weather
< windy, foggy weather
< exertion, in room
< apples; tobacco smoke

> open air

Arum triphyllum (2)

Sneezing < at night; much pricking in nose with **desire to bore** or pinch nose; dull, throbbing headache; sneezing without relief; soreness of nostrils; **acrid**, **excoriating discharge**, raw sores; **nose obstructed**, **breathes through mouth**; water, blood streaked discharge; pain at root of nose; scabs high up on right side of nose; **constant picking of nose until it bleeds**; face feels chapped; excessively cross and stubborn, **nervous**; raw cracked lips; hoarseness of voice; thirst but drinking causes pain; drowsiness; smarting of eyes; asthmatic breathing.

< overuse of voice
< talking; left side
< cold; wet winds

< heat; PM
< lying down

Arundo

Hayfever begins with burning and **itching in nostrils and roof of the mouth** (Wyethia); coryza, loss of smell (Nat m), sneezing **due to itching of nostrils**; burning and itching in auditory canals; eczema behind ears.

Dulcamara (2)

Constant sneezing; eyes swollen and watery leading to nose running and eyes swell again; **nose stuffs up with a cold rain**; nose completely stopped; thick, yellow mucus, bloody crusts; coryza of newborns; profuse watery lachrymation worse open air; granular lids; summer colds with diarrhea; aching in nose; **every cold settles in eyes**, throat or affects bladder; frequent urination; thirst; **chilly**.

< being chilled; **while hot**	> moving about
< sudden temperature changes	> external warmth
< cold, **wet**, feet, ground, cellars	
< cold bed	
< suppressions of sweat, discharges	
< eruptions	
< autumn; night; rest	
< before storms, injuries	

Euphrasia (2)

Much sneezing, **smarting lachrymation** and photophobia; bland nasal discharge; throat often involved with dry, hard cough; sore painful inner nose; **profuse fluent coryza**; **eyes water constantly**, blurring and swelling of lids, frequent blinking; sticky mucus on cornea; pressure in eyes; **catarrhal headache** with nasal discharge; thick yellow discharge from eyes; chronic sore eyes.

< sunlight, **wind**	> open air; winking
< warm room	> wiping eyes
< evening	> coffee; in dark
< lying down	

Gelsemium (2)

Violent sneezing; good at beginnings of the disease; summer colds; sneezing in AM; edges of nostrils red and sore; swallowing causes pain in ears; hot face; deafness; hands and feet are cold; colds due to weather changes; much tingling in nose; fullness at root of nose; dryness of nasal fossae; swollen turbinates; thin watery, excoriating discharge; concurrent dull headache and fever; **heavy dropping eyelids**; double vision; sensation as if hot water flowing from nose; **thirstless**, stuffy nose; chill runs up and down spine; colds from **warm** weather; headache with profuse urination.

< emotions, **dread**, surprise	> profuse urination
< shock; motion; **bad news**	> sweating; shaking
< weather, spring, humid, foggy muggy	> alcohol use; mental effort
< heat of summer	> bending forward
< dentition; tobacco; gas	> open air; stimulants
< before thunderstorms	
< thinking of ailments; 10 AM	

Natrum mur (3)

Violent, **fluent coryza**, lasts 1–3 days then stops up nose; loss of smell (Arundo); difficulty breathing; thin, watery discharge, **like raw white of egg**; **loss of smell and taste**; nose sore internally, dry, lachrymation of affected side, burning, acrid; swollen lids; sneezes early in AM; alternates fluent and dry coryza; hammering, heavy bursting headache over eyes; blue circles under eyes; **thirsty**; chilly.

< 9–11 AM; sun, alternate days	> open air, cool bathing
< heat; exertion, eyes, mental	> perspiration; rest
< violent emotions; music	> deep breathing; before breakfast
< sympathy; noise, warm room	> lying on right side; tight clothes
	> pressure in back

Nux vomica (1)

Prolonged sneezing spells; nose stuffed up at night; much irritation of nose, eyes and face; itching from larynx to trachea; face feels as if close to hot plate; **chilly**, **irritable**; **sniffles** after exposure to dry, cold; fluent coryza during day stuffed up at night; alternates between nostrils; bleeding in AM (Bry); photophobia < in AM; smarting, dry sensation of inner canthi; itching in ear through Eustachian tubes; sore nostrils; thirsty; dullness, oppression of frontal sinuses; scratchy sensation in throat; early stages.

< early AM	**> free discharges**
< cold, **open air**, drafts, wind	> naps; wrapping head
< uncovering	> rest; hot drinks
< high living, **coffee**, alcohol drugs	> milk; moist air
< sedentary habits	> evenings
< mental exertion; fatigue; vexation	> strong pressure
< disturbed sleep	
< noise; odors; touch; anger	
< pressure; clothes at waist	

Psorinum (3)

Boring, stinging in right nostril followed by excessive sneezing; burning followed by increased discharge which relieves; dry coryza with stoppage of nose; chronic postnasal drip; eyes-lids red, acrid secretion; **hungry or unusually well before an attack**; **anxiety**; profuse sweating; sensitive to drafts about head; **chilly**.

< cold, cold air, bathing	> lying with head low
< weather, changes, storms	> lying quietly; washing
< winter	> nosebleeds; hard pressure
< heat, of bed, exertion	> profuse sweating
< suppressions; coffee	> heat; warm clothing
< contact of his own limbs	
< least cold or draft	

Sabadilla (3)

Much itching of nose, **violent spasms of sneezing**; copious watery discharge from nose and eyes; severe frontal headache; **lachrymation** in open air and with bright lights; **redness of eyelids**; dry mouth with **no thirst**; muffled cough; tickling in nose spreads over entire body; sensitive smell; itching of soft palate; thirstless; craves hot things, sweets or milk; **chilly**.

< cold, air, drinks
< periodically, same hour,
< new moon, full moon
< odors, forenoon

> open air; heat
> eating, swallowing
> wrapped up

Sinapis nigra (3)

Mucus from posterior nares feels cold; scanty, **acrid** discharge; **stoppage of left nostril all day**, afternoon, evening, dry, hot lachrymation, sneezing; hacking cough > lying down; **nostrils alternating stopped up**; thick, lumpy secretions.

Consider:

Kali bic (1)

Sneezing; fluid, acrid discharge; excoriating mucous membrane from nose to throat; pinching pain across bridge of nose > with hard pressure; snuffles in children; **pressure and pain at root of nose**; **ulcerated septum**; **thick**, **ropy**, **greenish yellow discharge**, difficult to get out; **tough**, **elastic plugs in nose**; **loss of smell** (Arund, Nat m); **violent sneezing**; chronic inflammation of frontal sinuses; eyelids burn, swollen; **ropy**, yellow discharge; **aching and fullness in glabella**, thirsty, **chilly**.

Kali iod (2)

Incessant sneezing for an hour or more every AM; aching, heavy pressure between eyes; **copious watery discharges**, **acrid**, salty, thick or thin,hot, green, foul; puffy eyes; acrid coryza with dyspnea, salivation; colds from damp days; thirsty.

Silicea (2)

Nose cold sets in with itching, tingling, violent sneezing; itching and irritation of posterior nares or Eustachian tubes, causing patient to swallow to relieve; itching at point of nose; dry hard crust form which **bleed when loosened**; sneezing in AM; obstruction with loss of smell; frothy nasal discharges; coryza with epistaxis, **chilly**, **thirsty**.

Sticta (2)

Feeling of fullness at root of nose; dryness of nasal membranes; constant need to blow nose but no discharge; dry scabs, in AM and PM; incessant sneezing; **hay fever, catarrhal headache before discharge appears**; burning and soreness of eyes; eyelids; throat raw; **dry hacking cough at night, inspiration.**

Wyethia

Dryness of throat and pharynx with difficulty in swallowing; desires to swallow constantly with difficulty in clearing throat; intense itching of roof of mouth (Arundo) and posterior nares; sensation as if throat is swollen.

Symptoms in Kent's Repertory	**Page**
Eye, Lachrymation, coryza during	245
Nose, Catarrah, extends to frontal sinuses	324
Nose, Coryza, air, open, agg./amel.	326
Nose, Coryza, annual	326
Nose, Coryza, violent attacks	329
Nose, Discharge, copious	330
Nose, Discharge, crusts, scabs inside	330
Nose, Discharge, excoriating	331
Nose, Discharge, watery	333
Nose, Discharge, yellow	333
Nose, Discharge, posterior nares	333
Nose, Epistaxis, blowing the nose from	337
Nose, Obstruction, sensation of	341
Nose, Obstruction, warm room	341
Nose, Pain, root	344
Nose, Pain, inside/septum	347
Nose, Smell, acute/sensitive to odors	349
Nose, Sneezing, frequent	351
Nose, Snuffles	351

HEADACHES

Headaches are commonly experienced by most everyone at some time during their life, though some people experience them more often than others. There are several different types of headaches. **Congestive** or **migraine headaches** are often preceded by a warning, are very painful, and may last for several days. **Tension** or **nervous headaches** are often associated with stress or emotional situations. **Sick headaches** are head pain caused by other conditions somewhere else in the body such as from a congested liver, poor kidney function, or digestive disturbances which lead to a buildup of toxins. **Hormonal headaches** are associated with endocrine system imbalances such as premenstrual syndrome or diabetes.

Headaches are not themselves a disease but rather an indication that there is a disturbance elsewhere. They are due to an increase in pressure inside the skull from a dilation of the blood vessels. This pressure causes pain which will be experienced differently by different people. Thorough case-taking is, therefore, necessary to determine how the condition affects the individual person.

Most headaches are caused by conditions that are not considered life-threatening but are often a reflection of some chronic disturbance that the person suffers from. In most cases, the person knows what has caused the headache. A headache that is persistent, extremely painful, or awakes the person at night and is not relieved by any self-treatments or over-the-counter medications needs to be assessed by a physician.

I. Congestive/Migraine

Apis (3)

Located in occiput and posterior neck; meningitis; throbbing; sensation of swelling and pressure, occipital pain travels to neck;

stinging; stabbing, burning pain; sharp cries; headache over eyes to vertex to occiput; pain through orbits; photophobia; whole brain feels **very tired**; **awkward**, **drops things**; heat, throbbing, distensive pains > on pressure; < motion; bores head into pillow, screams out; eye lids **swollen**, red; conjunctiva bright red, puffy; **rolls their head**.

< heat, **room**, weather, drinks, bed	**> cool**, **air**, bath uncovering
< hot bath; touch (even of hair)	> pressure, slight expectoration
< after sleep; 4 PM	
< motion; suppressed eruptions	
< touch, right side	

Belladonna (3)

Pulsating, throbbing; **comes and goes quickly**; more right sided; congested; jarring and noise are intolerable; hysteria > holding head in direction opposite from affected part; sensation as if pain pressing into forehead and disappears when head is held back; stiffness in occiput; sensation as if a knife stabbing in temple to other temple; **sudden onset**; blushed face, restless; red and hot, **throbbing**; motion will make headache < but patient continues to move due to pain; **fullness in forehead**; bores head into pillow; suddenly cries; constant moaning; ill effects from having hair cut; **head sensitive to cold**, **drafts**; **dilated pupils**; dry, hot mouth.

< heat; afternoon (3 PM)	> light cover
< drafts; on head, hair cut	> bending backward
< washing head; taking cold	> bed rest
< check sweat; **light**, **noise**	> firm pressure
< jarring; touch, company	> standing, sitting
< pressure; motion, hanging down	

Bryonia (3)

Bursting frontal headache, as if it would split apart; **sensation of pressure on or above left eye or temple**; **thirsty**; feels sick with attempts to sit up; **pain always shifts to side lain on**; **congestive**; mental dullness and confusion; head feels full and wants to tie it up or press on it; **must keep perfectly still**, **quiet**; insidious onset; throbbing, not felt until they move; feels as if hit with a hammer from within; becomes seated in occiput; drawing in of bones toward zygoma; **faintness**, **vertigo on rising up**; **thirst for large drinks**; **full quick hard pulse**.

< motion; **rising up**; **stooping**	**> firm pressure**; **lying on painful part**
< coughing deep breathing	**> cool open air**; **quiet**
< dry, cold, heat	> cloudy, damp days
< becomes hot; warm room, weather	> drawing knees up
< eating; acids; light	> heat to inflamed parts
< vexation; touch; taking cold	> closing eyes; rest
< early AM, suppressions	
< opening eyes	

Gelsemium (3)

Hypertension; congested from flu; **sensation of pressure and blurred vision**; eye strain; occipital pain to trapezius; tension, stress; **sensation as if band wrapped around head**; heaviness of eyelids, limbs; blindness before headache; wants to be still with head raised; **no thirst**; vertigo spreading from occiput; bruised sensation; **pain in temple extending into ear**; muscle soreness of neck, shoulders; scalp sore to touch; delirious on falling to sleep; **confused**; ciliary neuralgia; bursting pains in eyes from occiput.

< emotions; **dread**; **shock**	> profuse urination
< motion; dentition; 10 AM	> sweating
< spring, **humid weather**, foggy, muggy	> shaking head, alcohol
< heat of summer, tobacco; gas	> mental effort
< before a thunderstorm	> raising head; open air
< thinking of ailments	> bending forward
	> continued motion
	> stimulants

Glonoine (3)

Vascular arterial **throbbing**, follows heat or sun stroke; **upward surges of blood** in forehead synchronous with pulse; crushing weight across forehead; pulsations from forehead to vertex; holds head, presses forehead; warm weather onset; **confusion** with dizziness;

heavy head but cannot lie on pillow; **cannot bear any heat around head**; very irritable; head feels large as if skull was too small; headache increases and decreases with sun; headache in place of menses; pains in malar bones (cheek) ending in headache; sharp shooting pain behind ears; veins of temples swollen; heat on crown of head; heat with hot sweat; scalp becomes sore due to the pain; vertigo with headache, patient has difficulty keeping head erect.

< heat, **on head**, **sun**, **weather**	> open air; elevating head
< motion, **shaking**, **jar**; injury	> cool things; stillness
< bending head back; left side	> cold applications, bathing
< wine; suppressed menses; fruits	> brandy; pressure; lying
< weight of hair, hair cut	
< stimulants; lying down	
< 6 AM to noon	

Helleborus niger (3)

Sensorial (mental) **depression**; stupefying headache; **rolls head** day and night; moaning, sudden screaming; **bores head into pillow**; beats head with hands; dull pain in occiput with sensation of water swishing inside; headache ends with vomiting; eyes turn upwards; slow to answer; **involuntary sighing**; aggravated 4–8 PM (Lyc); gradual onset of headache; numbing headache; hydrocephalus, stupid staring or tired look; face is pale; **thirsty**.

< cold air; puberty	> strong attention
< dentition; exertion	
< suppressions; uncovering	
< evenings (4–8 PM) to mornings	

Ipecac

Headache with nausea and vomiting, patient wishes to lie down which does not ameliorate the symptoms; **wants to vomit but can not** (Nux v) and ***is not > from vomiting if they are able;*** pain centers behind the eyes, through the eye balls; much lachrymation and **photophobia**; heavy, bruised feeling of the skull; blue rings around eyes; patient is **irritable**, short and adverse to light and noise; (Tabaccum has more nausea than Ipecac); thirsty, chilly.

< lying down; light; noise

Lachesis (3)

Most often left side; **pain comes in waves of deep pain at root of nose**, **temple**, **whole left side**; pressure and burning at vertex; pain through head on waking; bursting, surging pain, pulsation from head to foot; sensation as if all blood was in head; pain < after moving; sun headaches; dim vision, flickering, pale face, vertigo; eyes feel drawn together by knot at root of nose; **headache from suppressed menses**; **left side complaints move to right**; **loquacity**; headache moves down nose, right side feels cut off; **must loosen collar**; thirsty, chilly.

< after sleep, AM	**> open air**
< heat, **sun**, **room**, **drinks**	**> discharges**
< swallowing, **empty**, liquids	> hard pressure
< suppressed discharges, cloudy weather	**> cold drinks**; bathing parts
< climaxis, **alcohol**,	> warm applications
< start and close of menses; closing eyes	
< lying; motion; warm bath	
sensitive to, **slight touch**; **clothes**, noise	

Lycopodium (3)

Headache over eyes; long-standing coryza; hepatic, renal pathology, gout; pressure at vertex; may come and go after laughing; right vertical hemianopsia; connected with gastric complaints, if a meal is missed (Cact); prolonged throbbing, congestive, as if head would burst; pain in temples as if screwed together; headache from lying down, stooping; headache over eyes in severe colds; tearing occipital pain; deep furrows on forehead; shakes head without apparent cause; repeating or alternating symptoms; **awakes angry**; pain travels to opposite side where it is worse; **much gas**.

< pressure of clothes	**> warm drinks**, food
< warmth; awaking; wind	> cold applications; motion
< eating; to satiety; oysters	> urinating; eructations
< indigestion; **4–8 PM**	**> motion**; after midnight
< right side; from right to left	> being uncovered
< warm applications except around throat	

Melilotus (3)

Mean, bursting headache **through entire head**; sick headache; sensation as if brain will burst through head; injected conjunctiva, red eyes; headache > with epistaxis **and menses**, < after noon and coition; unable to fix mind; retching and vomiting; sense of pressure over orbits; pallor, cold hands and feet; black spots before eyes; **frontal throbbing**; undulating sensation in brain; eyes heavy, sight blurred, wants them closed tightly for relief; **neuralgia** around and over right side of head and neck; scalp sore tender to touch; **fiery red face**.

< climacteric; walking
< weather, changes, rainy, stormy
< motion; 4 PM

> bleeding; vinegar
> profuse urination

Natrum mur (2)

Blinding headache; sensation as if a **thousand little hammers knocking on brain**; blurred vision and vision changes; tend to throb and persist especially at 10 AM, 3 PM; disturbed by excitement; zigzag and flickerings around eyes; head feels too large; cold; anemic headache in school children; nervous, discouraged, broken down; chronic headaches, semilateral, congestive, from sunrise to sunset, pale face, nausea, vomiting; from eyestrain, menstrual; before an attack, numbness and tingling in lips, tongue and nose; headache > sleep; **pain in eyes when looking down**; thin, thirsty, hopeless, **dryness**, emaciation, headaches < reading, < motion, > pressure on eyes, chilly.

< 9–11 AM; sun; after menses
< alternate days; **heat**
< talking
< exertion, eyes, mental
< violent emotions; sympathy
< puberty; lying; noise
< music; seashore

> open air; cool bathing
> sweating; rest; before breakfast
> deep breathing
> lying on right side
> going without regular meals
> pressure against back
> tight clothing

Phosphorus (3)

Chronic head congestion; sensitive to all external impressions, odors, noise, touch; congestive, throbbing, sudden onset; face flushed and hot; burning pains; brain fag with **coldness of occiput**; vertigo with faintness; skin of forehead feels too tight; head heavy, aches over one eye; desires cold drinks.

< lying on left or painful side; **back**	> eating; sleep
< emotions; talking; touch	> cold, food, water to face
< odors; night	> being rubbed
< cold, **hands**, open air	> sitting up; in dark
< warm ingesta	
< sexual excesses; ascending stairs	
< weather changes, windy, cold, thunderstorms	
< AM and PM; mental fatigue	

Sanguinaria (3)

Right side and radiates from occiput and settles above right eye where it remains; awake in AM with headache (Lac defloratum, right eye to right occiput); headache < during the day, > at night; **circular red cheeks, flushed**; toxic feeling; sensitive to smells, noise; **veins and temples are distended**; pain > lying down and sleep; pain in small spot over left parietal bone; burning eyes; pain like flash of lightening; headaches every 7th day (Sabad, Sulph) climacteric; irritable, grumbles; red burning cheeks; has hot feet and hands which they stick out of the covers at night.

< periodically, **with sun**, weekly	**> sleep**; lying on back
< night; odors; jar; climaxis	> vomiting; urination
< light, looking up, raising arms	> passing gas; cool air
< sweets; right side; touch; motion	> acids; darkness

Sulphur (3)

Awakes with it; inactivity; eyes red, often with lachrymation, nausea and vomiting; head feels stupid, cannot think; bright red face; constant **heat on top of head** (Cupr, Graph); heaviness, fullness; pressure in temples; beating headaches < stooping, with vertigo; periodic sick headache; heat, **burning in eyes**; **lid margins red**; forgetful, averse to business; childish, peevish; irritable, thin, < standing; hot head, cold feet; sensation as if a band about (Gels) or deep pain in brain; **hungry**; **thirsty**, chilly.

< suppressions; speaking	> open air; motion
< bathing; milk; standing	> warm applications, weather
< atmospheric changes; rest	> sweat; dry heat
< heated, **in bed**, **exertion**	> lying on right side
< 11 AM; full moon, climacteric	> drawing up affected limbs
< alcohol; periodically	

Consider:

Aconite (2)

Rapid onset; sensation of heat/warmth; bursting **intracranial pressure**; associated with vertigo, rapid weather changes; much throbbing in temples, on one side then other; restless, **thirsty**, sensitive; > lying quietly in dark.

Arnica (3)

After trauma; **hot**, **with cold body**; confused; brain is sensitive with sharp, pinching pains; scalp feels contracted; cold spot on forehead; brain feels tired; says they aren't sick.

Iris — See sick headache.

Onosmodium

Vertigo, and sinus headaches; great affinity around eyes; eye strain brings it on; decreased sexual desire; temporal, mastoid, occipital to frontal; **mostly left-sided**; eye pain; tight ocular muscles; feel heavy, blurred vision; memory loss; dull, heavy, dizzy, pressing upward in occiput; > undressed; cold drinks, lying on back; < tight clothes, jarring.

Prunus

Shooting pain from right frontal bone through brain to occiput; **pain in right eye as if it would burst**.

Spigelia

Left-sided sinus headache; above left eye, frontal, temporal; nasal catarrh and postnasal drip; **pain beneath frontal eminence and temples, extending to eyes**; violent, painful throbbing; pain as if band around head; **very sensitive to touch**.

Veratrum viride

Acute congestive hyperemia; hot and heavy; markedly **dilated pupils**; delirious; diplopia; can develop meningitis; bloated, livid face; **pain from nape of neck**; Hippocratic face; sunstroke; **flushed face**; thirsty, cannot hold up head; double vision; **becomes faint on sitting up**.

II. Tension/Nervous Headaches

Agaricus (3)

Head in constant motion; dull headache from prolonged desk work; falling backward as if a weight in occiput; lateral headache as if from a nail (Coff, Ign); icy coldness, **like icy needles**, splinters; neuralgia with cold head; desires to cover head warmly (Hep, Sil); **nosebleed** with headache or thick mucous discharge; **vertigo from sunlight**, on walking; head **twitches, jerks**; headache > after stool or urine; nervous, restless; **uncertain, exaggerated motions**; spine sensitive, > touch, pressure; night sweats, sweats alternate sides; **double vision twitching of lids, eyes; fearlessness, loquacity; delirious**.

< air, **cold, freezing, open**
< stormy weather, before it
< mental exhaustion; coition
< alcohol; pressure; touch
< AM; menses
< pressure on dorsal spine which causes involuntary laughter

> gentle motion
> slow movement

Argentum nit (3)

Diarrhea and anxiety; brain and spinal symptoms; **trembling and coldness**; boring pain in left frontal region; emotional stresses; much excitement; **vertigo** is common; **sensation as if head is too**

large, as if bones in skull were separated; pain changes location; desires cold air and drinks; hemicranial attacks; memory weakness with debility; from mental exertion, dancing; aching in frontal eminence with **enlarged feeling of corresponding eye**; boring pain; scalp itches; blurred vision; head feels as if in a vice; 11–12 AM migraine; mental and digestive symptoms; **intolerance of heat**; **impulsive**, **hurried**; **melancholic**; **time passes slowly**; **craves sweets**; **thirsty**, chilly.

< emotions; **anxiety**; night	**> cold**, **air**, bath
< in room, sugar, shut in	> hard pressure; motion
< lying on right side; looking down	> eructations; fresh air
< drinking; crowds; warmth	
< cold food; **sweets**; menses	
< left side	

China (3)

Sensation as if skull would burst, as if brain balancing to and fro, striking against skull (Sulph, Sulph ac); intense **throbbing** of head and carotids; spasmodic headache at vertex with pain as if sides of head bruised; flushed face after hemorrhage, sexual excesses, loss of fluids; relieved from pressure and warm room; sensitive scalp; < touching hair; aches worse in open air, from temple to temple; dizziness with walking; blue color around eyes; **pressure in eyes**; spots before eyes; **nervous erethism** (abnormal irritability, sensitivity); apathetic; indifferent; disobedient; disposed to hurt others feelings; chilly; **thirsty**.

< loss of vital fluids; **touch**;	> hard pressure
< jar; alternate days; **periodically**	> loose clothes
< cold, drafts; wind; noise	> bending double
< open air; mental exertion	> open air
< eating; fruits; milk	> warmth
< night; **after eating**	
< bending over	

Coffea (3)

Coffee withdrawal; tight pain, < noise, odors, narcotics; brain seems as if torn to pieces, **as if nail were driven in head**; **sensitive**

hearing; acuteness of senses; irritable; easy comprehension; **excited**; **oversensitive**; **overactive**; **nervous sleeplessness**; rushing of ideas; resents sympathy; weeps; laments and tosses about; flushed face from rush of blood.

< noise; touch; odors	> lying; sleep; warmth
< open air; wind	> holding ice in mouth
< emotions; mental exertion	
< overeating, alcohol; night	
< narcotics; cold	> open air (headache)
< eating (headache)	

Ignatia (3)

Headache from grief, loss; much nervousness; acute hysteria; more psychosomatic; sensation as if a nail driven into head; intense pressure often over a small spot; inclines head forward, pain at root of nose; head feels hollow, heavy; **< stooping**, **< smoking or smelling tobacco**; headache ends in yawning and vomiting; enjoys being sad; **alert**, **oversensitive**, **nervous**; **sighs**, weeps or laughs; changes moods quickly; doesn't communicate; very sensitive; may be somewhat immature acting.

< emotions; **grief**, **worry**	> change of position
< shock; odors; touch; fright	> lying on affected part
< air, open, cold	> urination; pressure
< coffee; tobacco; liquids	> alone; while eating
< in AM; after meals	
< external warmth	

Kali phos (2)

Headache in overworked school children; stress from studying; lassitude and fatigue; increased sexual desire; occipital; > rising; vertigo from lying, on standing, sitting and looking up, **cerebral anemia**; headache with weary, empty, gone feeling in stomach (Ign, Sep); weakness of sight; **nervous**, **sensitive**, **easily fatigued**; **irritable**; starts easily; anxiety; depression; shyness; averse to their own; thirsty; **chilly**.

< excitement; worry; puberty	> sleep; eating
< mental fatigue; touch	> gentle motion

< pain; cold, dray air	> warmth
< physical exertion	> nourishment
< eating; early AM	

Phosphoric acid (3)

Will not eat; deep reacting remedy; becomes indifferent; exhausted; hair falls out; diabetes from grief; **crushing head pain** in area of temples and vertex; neurasthenia due to nervous exhaustion; may have vertigo; heavy head, **confused**, **pressure at vertex**; **vertigo towards evening**; **when standing or walking**; dull headache from eyestrain (Nat m), coition; **blue rings around eyes**; averse to sunlight; listless; **apathetic**, **indifferent**; effects of grief and shock; quiet; poor memory (Anac); **sleepy daytime**; profuse sweats; **chilly**; marked growth spurts in children.

< debility; **loss of fluids**	> warmth; short sleep
< sexual excesses; fatigue	> stool
< fever; convalescence	
< emotions; grief, shock	
< homesickness; chagrin; disappointed love	
< drafts; cold; music; talking	
< exertion	

Zincum met (3)

Nervous and exhausted; very restless, **especially feet and legs**; **occipital headache**; **hot occiput cool forehead**; weak memory; **very sensitive to noise**; averse to work, talk; head feels like it will fall to left side; headache from wine; rolls head from side to side; bores head into pillow; sensation of weight on vertex; overtaxed school children; starting in fright; **rolls eyes**, **squinting**; blurred half of vision; **child repeats everything said to it**; **lethargy**; **stupid**; screams if moved during sleep; varying intensity headache; heavy ache in temples, grinds teeth; hair painful; eyes feel drawn together; thirsty.

< exhaustion, mental	> motion; hard pressure
< suppressions; noise; touch	> warm open air
< wine; after being treated	**> free discharges**; eruptions
< menses; 5–7 PM	> eating
< after dinner	

Gelsemium (3)—See migraine

Natrum mur (3)—See migraine

Nux vomica (3)—See sick headaches

Phosphorus (3)—See migraine

Pulsatilla (3)—See hormonal

Consider:

Asafoetida (3)

Irritable; complains of trouble; **oversensitive**; boring pain above eyebrows; **pressive pain from within outward**; orbital neuralgia; pains associated with numbness; violent hard throbbing; > open air; > pressure.

Thuja (3)

Chronic nervous headaches in sycotic miasms.

III. Sick Headaches (caused by other symptoms)

Chelidonium

Liver-related headaches; **pains under right scapula** with pain at right eyebrow; icy coldness of occiput from nape of neck; **feels heavy as lead**; lethargic; marked **drowsiness** with general numbness; vertigo; inclined to fall forward; right-side headache behind ear and shoulder blade; **neuralgia over right eye**, cheekbone and ear; excessive lachrymation following liver pain; yellow sclera; orbital neuralgia with profuse tearing; sweaty with aversion to uncover and without relief; lazy, indisposed to move; thirsty; chilly.

< motion; cough; touch	> hot food; eating
< weather changes, 4 AM & PM	> milk; pressure; hot bath
< right side	> bending backward; after eating

Cocculus

Seasickness, car sick; persons taking care of terminally ill who get exhausted; nausea and vertigo; pain from **occiput** to nape of neck; **sense of emptiness in head**; cannot lie on back part of head; contracted pupils; sensation of opening and shutting, especially in occiput; head trembles; eye pain as if eye is torn out of head; facial nerve paralysis; **hollow feeling**; sensitive to cold; heavy head; occiput > bending backward; sadness, taciturn, peevish, easily offended; thirsty; chilly.

< motion; emotions; loss of sleep
< exertion; pain; touch; noise
< anxiety; cold, open air
< eating; menses; smoking; afternoons

Iris

Sick headache with nausea and vomiting associated with blurred vision; **especially from eating sweet things**; pain over eyes; periodic migraines; hypochlorhydria with burning in abdomen; averse to light; frontal headache; scalp feels constricted; right temple especially affected; headache < rest; begins with a blur before eyes, after relaxing from mental strain; **bilious**, **sour vomitus**, **burning**; diarrhea with headache.

< weekly; 2–3 AM	> gentle motion
< spring and fall; after midnight	
< mental exhaustion	
< hot weather; evening	
< from rest	> open air

Nux vomica

Indigestion; over-stimulation; over either eye or in occiput; after eating; urge to stool after eating, during headache and cannot; yellow/green tongue; sensation as if a nail driven through head; headache in AM; brain feels as if it is turning in a circle; **vertigo with momentary loss of consciousness**; pressing on vertex; sensitive scalp; frontal headache, with desire to press head against something; **headache in sun** (Glon, Nat c); feels distended and sore within; photophobia; **sensitive to noise**, **odors**, **light**; **irritable**; **sullen**; **impatient**; blood shot eyes; after tobacco, alcohol, overeating; **angry**; cannot stand pain; **chilly**; thirsty.

< **cold**; **open air**; drafts, wind	> free discharges; naps
< **uncovering**; **coffee**; **excesses**	> wrapping head; resting
< overeating; sedentary habits	> hot drinks; milk
< mental exertion; fatigue	> moist air; evening
< anger, noise, odors, light, touch	> strong pressure
< **pressure of clothes**	

Picric acid

Mental fatigue; prolonged mental strain; **neurasthenia**; **uremia**; cannot think anymore; **headache > with tight bandaging**; **occipital pain**; anxiety and dread of failure at examination; vertigo and noises in ears; boils **within ears** and back of neck; weakness; headache > nose bleed.

< exertion, mental or physical	> rest; cold; in sun
< seminal loss; heat	> bandaging; tight pressure
< after sleep; wet weather	> cold water

Sulphur

Sensation of heat at vertex (Cupr, Graph), pressure in temples; periodic sick headache; sensation of beating or throbbing; fullness; flushed face, cold feet; **constant heat at top of head**; heaviness; **dry scalp**; heat and **burning in eyes**; forgetful; difficult mentation; busy; irritable; sensation as if a band about or pains deep in brain; Sunday headaches; preceded by photopsia; sweaty scalp, dry hair; halo about a light; photophobia; swollen veins of forehead; **red orifices**, nose, eyes, mouth, anus; **suddenly hungry**,< 11 AM; chilly; **thirsty**; night sweats.

< **suppressions**; **bathing**; milk	> open air; motion
< **heated**, **exertion**, **in bed**	> warm applications
< atmospheric changes; speaking	> sweating; dry heat
< 11 AM; full moon; climacteric	> lying on right side
< rest; standing; alcohol	> drawing up affected limbs

Sanguinaria—See migraines

IV. Hormonal Headaches

Cyclamen

Similar to Pulsatilla, except is chilly; headache with menses; vertigo and visual disturbances either during or after menses; pain one sided; maybe either; aching in AM, with **flickering before eyes**; vertigo, things turn in a circle; better in the room; worse open air; one sided headache; brain feels wrapped up; pain in left temple; prolonged migraine; **flickering of various colors** before eyes; terrors of conscience; depression, with weeping, desire to be alone.

< cold; evening; fresh air
< sitting; fats
< cold water

> motion, during menses
> weeping; warm room
> rubbing parts; lemonade

Graphites

Rush of blood to head, flushed face also with nosebleed, distention and flatus; headache in AM on waking, mostly one side with inclination to vomit; sensation of cobweb on forehead, **headache during menses**; rheumatic pains on one side of head extending to teeth and neck; **burning on vertex** (Cupr, Sulph); **eyelids swollen and red**; **pains go to part lain on**; **weeps from music**; heaviness of occiput; timid, unable to decide; apprehensive, despondent; constipated; **over weight**; **chilly**; **costive**; laughs at reprimands; cracks and fissures of skin.

< cold, drafts; light
< menses, during and after
< suppressed eruptions
< empty swallowing; fats
< warmth of bed; night
< scratching; wet feet
< hot drinks

> open air
> eating; touch
> in dark
> wrapping up

Pulsatilla

Wandering pains; **right temporal**, may cause lachrymation, crying; headache before, during and **after cessation of menses**; pain goes to side lain on; decreased appetite and thirst; pains extend to face and teeth; frontal and supraorbital pains; **scalding lachrymation of affected side**; **headache from overwork**; pressure on vertex; cannot lie with head low; profuse scalp sweats; occipital ace, < coughing; **thirstless**; **timid**; **emotional**; **weepy**; **peevish**; likes sympathy.

< warmth, air, room, bed
< suppressions; **evening**; **rest**
< beginning motion; getting feet wet
< lying; on left side
< eating; **fats**; **rich foods**; ices
< puberty; pregnancy; before menses
< hanging feet down

> cold; **fresh**; **open air**
> uncovering; **erect posture**
> gentle motion; weeping
> consolation
> cold food and drink

Sepia

Sensation as if a band around head (Gels); during and after menses; nervous; pain over one eye; throbbing pain; stinging pain from within outward and upward, mostly left or in forehead, with nausea and vomiting; coldness of vertex; jerking of head backward and forward; headache in **terrible shocks** at menses, with scanty flow; **indifferent** to loved ones; averse to occupation, **family**; irritable, easily offended; dreads to be alone; **very sad**; weeps when telling symptoms; miserly; anxious toward evening; sensitive to pain; **feels cold**, even in a warm room; poor memory; hair loss; headache, over left eye; alternates sides, < lying on it; sensitive to odors; chilly.

< cold, **air**, wind, wet, snowy
< sexual excesses; before menses
< pregnancy; abortion
< AM and evenings, after first sleep
< before thunderstorms
< washing; left side; after sweat

> violent motion
> warmth; cold drinks
> cold bathing
> drawing limbs up
> pressure

Glonoine— See migraine

Lycopodium— See migraine

Natrum mur— See migraine

Consider:

Kreosotum

Dull pain as if from a board pressing against forehead; **menstrual headache**; occipital pain; dissatisfied, cross, obstinate; pressing outward pains, especially in the forehead; headache associated with drowsiness; > warmth; < rest, stooping and cold; **< before menses**.

Symptoms in Kent's Repertory	**Page**
Head, Pain, catarrhal	137
Head, Pain, cold, becoming from	138
Head, Pain, excitement of the emotions, after	139
Head, Pain, heated, from becoming	140
Head, Pain, mechanical injuries, after	141
Head, Pain, light in general/artificial	141
Head, Pain, mental exertion, from	143
Head, Pain, noise, from	144
Head, Pain, stooping	148
Head, Pain, straining eyes, from	149
Head, Pain, sun, exposure to	149
Head, Pain, warm room agg./amel.	151
Head, Pain, weather, from changes of/cold/damp	151
Vision, Flickering, headache, before/during	279
Stomach, Nausea, headache, during	508
Stomach, Vomiting, headache, during	533

HEAT STROKE/EXHAUSTION

Heat stroke is due to prolonged exposure to heat and sunlight which results in increased sweating and subsequent loss of fluids and electrolytes such as sodium, chloride and potassium. While the body is usually able to regulate the amount of fluid loss, in the elderly and very young this regulatory mechanism is incomplete, resulting in heat stroke. It is further compounded by the use of diuretics such as caffeine, prescription drugs or alcohol.

The condition often goes unnoticed by the person being affected until it is too late. The **first symptoms** may be confusion and fatigue which come and go and are followed by disorientation, agitation, loss of memory, violent behavior and collapse. The person's pulse may be rapid, respirations shallow and pupils constricted. There will be little perspiration and the skin will be hot and dry. If allowed to continue, the ultimate course is kidney and heart failure.

It is important that the person receive prompt medical attention, as heat stroke can progress rapidly, resulting in dehydration, shock and death.

Antimonium crud (3)

Pain in head from becoming heated, by a fire or stove; loss of voice from becoming overheated; **continual drowsiness in elderly**; unable to bear heat of sun, unable to work; **excessive irritability and fretfulness**; **thick coated white tongue**; peevish, **cannot bear to be touched, looked at**; aching headache, worse at vertex; eyes dull, sunken, red, agglutinated, **canthi raw and fissured**; redness of ears, swelling; nostrils **chapped and covered with crusts**; **yellow crusted eruptions on cheeks**, chin; **cracks at corners of mouth**; **voice harsh, badly pitched**; **urticaria**, measles-like eruptions of skin; no thirst; chilly; eyes sensitive to light; sensation of heat in face, especially cheeks.

< cold, **bathing**; **water**; **damp**	> open air; rest
< overeating, sweets	> moist warmth
< heat, summer sun, radiated	
< overheating; evenings	
< acids; wine	

Belladonna (3)

Head pain from becoming heated; rapid onset; flushed face; throbbing, burning head; **dilated pupils**; headache < stooping, moving; **no thirst**, **anxiety or fear**; delirium; convulsions; rages, strikes, **desires to escape**; **furious**; **acuteness of all senses**; eyes feel swollen, protruded, **staring**, **brilliant**; **dry**; **great thirst for cold water**, **dread of drinking**; abdomen distended, hot, very sensitive to touch; carotids throb; dry mouth with no thirst (Puls), skin **hot**; burning and dry; sweats only on covered parts; sweat with or after the heat; pulse full, bounding or rapid but weakened; **alternate redness and paleness of skin**; **bright red**, **glossy skin**; skin hot but moistness and dryness alternates; thirsty.

< heat, of sun, if heated	> light covering
< afternoon, 3 PM	> bending backward
< drafts; on head; washing head	> bed rest; semi-erect
< checked sweat; **light**; **noise**	
< jarring; touch; pressure	
< company; hanging down	

Bryonia (2)

Head pain from becoming heated; **dryness of mucous membranes**; **parched lips**, **dry**, **cracked**; **excessive thirst**; lips swollen, dry, cracked; **physical weakness**, **debility**; **very irritable**; wants to go home; painful feeling of fullness in head, **bursting splitting** headache, as if everything wants to come out; dryness of throat, sticking or swallowing, < coming into a warm room; **averse to least motion**; **dizziness or faintness with rising up**; **bitter taste** in mouth; **full**, **quick**, **hard pulse**; **excessive thirst for large quantities**; dyspepsia from heat; sensitive to touch; cough < in warm room (Nat c); **joints red**, **swollen**, **hot**; skin hot, painful; **thirsty**.

< motion, **stooping**, **exertion**	**> pressure**, **lying on**

< hot weather
< dry heat, cold
< hot, becoming, room
< drinking while hot; **eating**
< vexation; touch
< early AM

painful side
> cool, open air; **quiet**
> drawing knees up
> heat to inflamed part

Carbo veg (3)

Headache from becoming heated; vertigo with slightest movement of head; with nausea; patient seems lifeless but head is hot; pulse imperceptible, quickened respiration; must have air; wants to be fanned; head feels heavy; face pale, cold with cold sweat; Hippocratic faces, mottled cheeks and red nose, lips cracked; quivering of eyelids; heat pressure and burning pains in eyes; cannot bear tight clothing around abdomen; deep, rough, **hoarse** voice, fails on slight exertion; skin **blue**, **cold**, **ecchymosed**; marbled with venous distention; moist skin; **hot perspiration**; general itching < with becoming warm; thirsty, chilly; sudden memory loss.

< warmth; **depletions**
< cooling off; old age; evening
< high living; dissipation
< pressure of clothes
< over lifting; walking in open air
< fat food; coffee; milk; wine
< warm damp weather
<weather, extreme, cold night air
< wind on head

> eructations; cool air
> elevating feet
> from being fanned

Gelsemium

Dizziness, drowsiness, dullness, trembling; motor paralysis, great prostration; general depression from heat of sun; **muscular weakness**; slow pulse; depressed from heat; not from immediate effects of sun; heat exhaustion; dilation of pupils, dim sight; **apathy regarding condition**; lack of fear; desires to be quiet, left alone; heaviness of head, **dullness** of head; headache preceded by blindness; > profuse urination; wants head raised on pillow; face **hot**; **heavy**, **besotted look**; dusky hue of face; low jaw drooping; pulse soft, weak, full and flowing; slow when quiet but accelerated with motion; hot, dry, itching, measle like eruption of skin; **tremor**, **confusion**; less restlessness than Aconite and **less** violent onset than Belladonna; patient doesn't move due to weakness, not because it aggravates like Bryonia; **thirstless**.

< emotions; surprise; **dread**	> profuse urination
< shock; motion	> sweating; shaking
< weather, **spring**, **humid**	> alcohol; mental effort
< heat; tobacco; gas	> bending forward
< before a thunderstorm	> open air; continued motion
< thinking of ailments	

Glonoine (3)

Head pain from becoming heated; **by a fire or stove**; loss of senses, sinking down unconsciousness; nausea, vertigo, violent headache, flushed face and cold body, **surging of blood to head and heart**; **sensation of pulsations throughout body**; **confusion**; **heavy head but cannot lay it on pillow**; **throbbing** headache; sun headache; very irritable; reddened conjunctiva; mist, black spots, sparks before eyes; sees everything half light, half dark; ears throb, feel full; flushed, hot, livid, pale face, sweaty; face sunken or bloated and red; bluish face; swollen veins in temples; heavy tongue; full, tense pulse; heat with hot sweat; oppressed breathing, sighing; jaws firmly clenched; constriction and anxiety; violent, laborious action of heart; palpitations; great prostration; loss of sense of location.

< heat, **on head**, overheating	> open air; elevating head
< sun; hot weather; **open fire**	**> cool things**, **bathing**
< motion; **jarring**, bending head	> brandy
< wine; fruits; weight of hat	
< lying down; 6 AM to noon; left side	

Natrum mur (2)

Headache from becoming heated (Opium); hot weather fatigues, makes him languid, dizzy and faint; feels dull, sleepy, cannot work; vision is unsteady; **dry mucous membranes**; **great weakness and weariness**; head throbs; **eye muscles feel weak and stiff**, sees sparks; fiery zigzag appearance around objects; burning in eyes; lids swollen;

pain in eyes with looking down; lips and corners of mouth dry, ulcerated, cracked; **coldness of legs** with congestion to head; **numbness and tingling** in fingers, extremities; thirst moderate or drinks large quantities.

< 9–11 AM; with sun	> open air; cool bathing
< heat, sun; summer	> sweating; rest
< exertion; sympathy	> deep breathing
< violent emotions; noise	> lying on right side; pressure against back
< lying down	> tight clothing
< music; warm room	

Opium (2)

Head pain from becoming heated (Nat m); skin is hot and damp; **very hot, sweltering perspiration; except to lower limbs**; high temperature with intense thirst, **sleepiness without sleep**; complaints appear with perspiration; lack of vital reaction, **painlessness**; loquacious delirium, with open eyes and red face; fright with fear; heat in head with convulsions; eyes burning; hot, dry; face red, hot, **puffy**; red eyes half shut; dilated pupils and insensible; foaming at mouth; cold sweat on forehead; heaviness of head; pupils dilated; eyes staring, pupils fixed; face pale, earthy, red spots on cheeks; swollen veins of face; trembling of facial muscles; swollen lips; mouth dry with violent thirst; **paralysis of tongue**; involuntary urination or defecation; pulse irregular, unequal, **slow and full**, **complete loss of consciousness**; coma.

< emotions; **fear**; fright	> cold; uncovering
< joy; odors	> constant walking
< alcohol; sleep	> coffee
< suppressed discharges	
< if heated	
< during and after sleep	

Consider:

Aconite (2)

Headache from becoming heated; **physical and mental restlessness; sudden onset**; complaints **from very hot weather**; **great fear**, **anxiety**; eyes feel **hot**, **dry**; lids **swollen**, **red**; hot, red, flushed, swollen face; one cheek red, the other pale; skin red, hot, **dry**, burning; formication and numbness of skin; heart rate increases at first then decreases.

Amyl nitrite

Congestive stage of sunstroke; **anxiety**; longing for fresh air; **surging of blood to head and face**; **flushing followed by sweat**; sensation as if blood would start through skin; **tumultuous action of heart**; flushes of heat sometimes followed by cold and clammy skin; trembling hands; unsteady gait; tired feeling in legs.

Kali carb (2)

Sweating, **backache**, **weakness**; **pulse weak**, **rapid**, **intermittent**; burning in skin; **back and legs give out**; often seen in elderly who are dark-haired, of pale complexion and obese; may have difficulty perspiring and can have weakness of groups of muscles; may have a sense of fear in epigastrium.

Lachesis

Loquacity; delirium; weak memory; vertigo; glimmering before eyes; unable to tolerate extremes of temperature; face sunken or bloated, red; tongue paralyzed, trembles if protruded; constriction of throat; heart palpitations; feels constricted.

Lycopodium (3)

Tongue dry, black, cracked, swollen; blisters on tongue; dry throat without thirst; dry skin; **head pain from becoming heated**.

Silicea (2)

Headache from becoming heated; heat causes nausea, gastric ailments; gloominess, vertigo, unsteady and confused in actions; dry hard crusts which bleed; cracked skin.

Symptoms in Kent's Repertory	Page
Mind, Confusion during the heat	15
Mind, Delirium, raging, raving	19
Mind, Excitement, heat, during	40

Mind, Fear, of death 44
Mind, Speech, incoherent 81
Head, Sunstroke....................................... 231
Generalities, Heated, becoming (agg.) 1367
Generalities, Sun, exposure to......................... 1404
Generalities, Weakness, heat, from/of the sun 1417

HEMORRHAGES

Hemorrhage or blood loss may occur for a variety of reasons and may not always be visible. **Internal blood loss** shows as a weak, rapid pulse with shallow breathing and cold, clammy skin. There may also be tenderness over the affected area, restlessness and anxiety. The person may complain of dizziness or faintness.

External blood loss may occur from an artery or vein. **Arterial** blood flow will show as a spurting, pulsating flow of bright red blood, whereas **venous** flow will show as a darker red and steady, oozing flow.

Any **bleeding condition constitutes a medical emergency** and needs to be seen by a physician or emergency medical technician. Applying tourniquets or the application of direct pressure should be done in addition to treating with homeopathic medicines.

Arnica (3)

Affects stasis of venous system, ecchymosis, **hemorrhages** relaxed blood vessels; black and blue spots; bruises; thrombosis; hematocele; retinal hemorrhages; nasal bleeding after cough; blood from ears; vomiting of blood; uterine bleeding after damage from coitus; pulse feeble; irregular **tendency to hemorrhage**; **after trauma**; feels sore; bruised; thirsty.

< injuries, **bruises**, shock, sprains
< touch; after sleep; motion
< overexertion; jarring; labor
< rest; wine; damp cold

> lying; **head low**; outstretched

Belladonna

Bright, gushing, offensive; sudden onset; **nose bleeds** with red face, coryza, mucus mixed with blood; hematuria where no pathology found; increased menses flow; **bright red**, **early**; **profuse**; **hot**; rapid weakened pulse; throbbing pulse, carotids; **no thirst**; **anxiety or fear**.

< heat, of sun; afternoon (3 PM)	> light covering; bed rest
< drafts, on head, hair cut	> bending backward
< washing head; taking cold	> semi erect
< check sweat; **light**; **noise**; **jarring**	
< touch; company; motion	
< hanging down	

Bothrops (3)

Blood does not coagulate; **bleeds from body orifices**; from thrombosis; much lassitude; sluggishness; blindness from retinal hemorrhages; vomits black blood; intense hematemesis; black stools.

< right side

Cantharis (3)

Sudden loss of consciousness with red face; blood streaked **tenacious mucus**; vomits blood streaked membrane, violent retching; stools bloody with **burning and tenesmus**; **shuddering**; urine, bloody and comes drop by drop; menses early and profuse; **violent acute inflammation**; thirsty.

< urinating; drinking; cold	> warmth; rest
< bright objects; sound of water	> rubbing
< touch	

Carbo veg (3)

Stagnated blood, blueness, coldness, ecchymosis; decreased vital force from loss of fluids; hemorrhages from any mucous surface; **needs to be fanned**; face is cyanotic, puffy, pale, Hippocratic, cold sweat; **epistaxis daily with pale face**; nose bleeds with straining; blood oozes from gums with cleaning of teeth; discharge of blood from rectum; hemorrhage from lungs; purpura, **varicose ulcers**; **blueness of skin**; blood does not coagulate; dark oozing blood; thirsty, chilly.

< fats; butter; coffee; milk
< warmth; **depletions**,
< exhausting diseases; old age
< rich foods; **high living**; evening
< dissipation; walking in open air
< pressure of clothes; air, wind or head
< weather, cold night air, humid, frosty, extreme; cooling off

> eructations; cool air
> elevating feet
> from being fanned

China (3)

Bleeds from body orifices; passive hemorrhages; from slightest causes; **intermittent**; **profuse**; **exhausting hemorrhages**, bleeds easily from nose, especially on rising; early menses; **dark clots and abdominal discomfort**; profuse menses with pain; hemorrhages from lungs; **extreme sensitiveness to touch but hard pressure relieves**; oversensitive; nervous; better bending double; dark, foul, watery **bloody stool**, painless; **drenching night sweats**; **periodicity**; **thirst**; chilly.

< touch; **vital fluid loss**
< periodically; night
< cold; drafts, wind; noise
< open air; eating; fruit; milk
< mental exertion; **after eating**
< bending over

> hard pressure; open air
> loose clothing; warmth
> bending double

Crotalus h (3)

Passive oozing of blood; will not clot; **oozes from body orifices**; dark hemorrhages with no clotting; very sensitive to light; **absorption of intraocular hemorrhages**; non-inflammatory retinal hemorrhages; blood oozes from ears; epistaxis of **black**, **stringy** blood; cancer of tongue with bleeding; vomiting of blood, black, coffee ground vomitus; slimy mucus vomiting; with cancer of stomach; cannot tolerate clothing around epigastrium (Lach, Nux v); rectal bleeding; dark, oozes when standing or walking, coffee ground appearance; prolonged menses; dark, bloody urine; feeble, tremulous pulse; bloody expectoration; bloody sweat; **purpura**; blood boils which fill with dark fluid from blood and will break from overfilling or slightest touch; exudate is acrid, scalding; bleeds through pores of skin and under nails.

< lying on right side; AM & PM	> light; motion
< falling asleep; alcohol; awaking	
< warm weather; spring, open air; jarring	

Ferrum phos (2)

Bright hemorrhages from any orifice; vomits bright red blood, epistaxis; watery, bloody, frequent, stools with undigested food; hemoptysis bright red, especially in pneumonia; **short**, **quick**, **soft pulse**; thirsty.

< night (4–6 AM); noise	> cold; bleedings
< motion, cold air; jarring	> lying down
< checked sweat	
< right side	

Hamamelis (3)

Bleeds from slightest causes, oozing; venous congestion; painful varicose veins; **hemorrhoids**, with **bruised soreness of affected part**; vessels greatly injected; profuse epistaxis, passive flow, with tightness in ridge of nose; hematemesis of black blood; hematuria with much desire; uterine hemorrhage; menses **dark**, **profuse with sore abdomen**; hemoptysis with tickling cough; phlebitis; milk leg; ecchymosis with soreness; **soreness**.

< injury; bruises; pressure
< air; open, cold, humid
< motion; jar; touch

Ipecac (3)

Bright red, **gushing hemorrhages which clot quickly**; **continued nausea**; **no thirst**; epistaxis; vomits blood; uterine hemorrhage with **nausea**; **bright red**, **gushes**; bleeds from lungs, nausea; hemoptysis from slightest exertion, chilly.

< warmth, damp, room	> open air
< overeating, rich foods, ices, veal	
< periodically; moist warm wind	
< heat and cold; lying down	

Lachesis (3)

Blood will not clot; bleeds from body orifices; purpura; **loquacity**; nostrils bleed, are sensitive; swollen gums, bleed easily, spongy; bowel hemorrhages of **black particles**, charred straw; cyanosis; skin appears **bluish**, **purple**; purpura with prostration; **sleep into aggravation**; **fetor**; rapid onset; symptoms move from left to right.

< after sleep; AM; **heat**
< warm drinks; **swallowing**, **empty**
< slightest touch, **of clothes**, **around neck**
< retarded discharges;cloudy weather
< alcohol; left side; closing eyes

> open air; **free secretions**
> hard pressure; bathing part
> cold drinks
> warm applications

Melilotus (3)

Congestion; hemorrhages; **sick headache** > with epistaxis or **menses**; **profuse epistaxis**; red face; throbbing carotids; scanty menses; hemoptysis.

< climacteric; walking
< weather, changes, stormy, rain
< motion; 4 PM

> bleeding; profuse urination
> vinegar

Mercurius (3)

Streaked, stringy hemorrhages; bloody emissions, which do not relieve; bloody discharge from ears; nose bleeds at night; bloody salivation, metallic taste; gums spongy, receding and easily bleed; **great thirst for cold with moist mouth**, fetid breath; stools, **greenish**, **slimy and with blood**; bloody, albuminous urine; whooping cough with nosebleeds; **profuse perspiration with no relief**.

< night, night air
< sweating; **lying on right side**
< heated, in bed or from fire
< drafts to head
< weather changes; damp, cold
< heat and cold; wet feet

> moderate temperatures

Millefolium (3)

Acute onset bleeding; bright red blood; **epistaxis**, **bloody urine**; bleeding hemorrhoids and bloody stools; uterine hemorrhages of **bright red blood**; hemoptysis, with cough; bruised soreness; profuse, painless bright red fluid hemorrhage.

< injury; violent exertion	> bleeding; discharges

Nitric acid (3)

Blood does not coagulate; **epistaxis**, with chest affections; **bloody saliva**; profuse bright hemorrhage from bowels, easily bleeding hemorrhoids; urine is bloody, albuminous, smells like horses; uterine bleeds; early menses, profuse, like muddy water; bleeding after D & C; **irritable**; **hateful**; **sharp sticking pains**; **cracks and fissures**; **corrosive discharges**, offense; thirst; **chilly**; **perspires easily**.

< slight, **touch**; **jarring**; noise	> gliding motions; ridings
< motion; milk; after meals	> mild weather
< cold; air, damp	> steady pressure
< night; evening; hot weather	
< weather changes; heat of bed	
< mental exertion, shock	

Phosphorus (3)

Blood does not coagulate; **bleeds easily from orifices**; thrombosis of retinal vessels; **epistaxis rather than menses**; chronic catarrh with **small hemorrhages, polypi bleed easily**; gums **bleed easily**, persistent bleeding after tooth extraction; blood discharged from rectum during stool, hemorrhoids which bleed; hematuria, especially with Bright's disease; slight uterine hemorrhages between menses; repeated hemoptysis; **wounds bleed a lot even if small**, heal and break out again; petechiasis, ecchymosis, **purpura hemorrhages**; dreams of bleeding; oversensitive; polycythemia; fear of death when alone; blood streaked discharges of ulcers; **craves cold drinks**.

< lying on left side, painful side, back	> eating; sleep
	> cold, food, water to face
< emotions; talking; touch; odors; light	> rubbing; sitting up
	> in dark

< cold, **hands**; open air
< warm ingesta; salt
< weather, changes windy, cold
< thunderstorms; AM & PM
< mental fatigue
< ascending stairs

Sabina (3)

Bright red blood, **fluid and clots together**; hemorrhoids with much bleeding; bloody urine, much urging; **profuse**, **bright menses**; discharge of blood between periods, with sexual excitement, hemorrhages, worse from **least motion**; see postpartum bleeding.

< nightly; pregnancy; climacteric
< heat; bed, room, exercise
< foggy weather
< least motion

> cold; cool; open air

Secale (3)

Blood does not clot; oozes, thin, fetid, watery black blood; **nosebleeds**, dark, oozing; tongue dry, **cracked**, **blood like ink exudates**; vomits coffee ground, bloody fluid; **unnatural ravenous appetite**, **unquenchable thirst**; stools **olive green**, **thin**, **putrid**, **bloody**; discharge of black blood from bladder; passive uterine hemorrhages; skin, bluish color, easily bleeding wounds, petechiasis, **skin feels cold to touch** but will not tolerate covering; varicosities; passive bleeding or discharges; **internally is hot**; **burning**; **externally is cold**; See post partum hemorrhage; **thirsty**.

< warmth; during menses
< pregnancy
< loss of fluids
< covers

> cold, bathing, uncovering
> rocking; rubbing
> forcible extension of limbs

Sulphuric acid (3)

Hemorrhages, violent, **black**, thin; **tremor and weakness**, especially in elderly; **purpura hemorrhagica**; **intra-ocular hemorrhage after trauma**; aphthae; gums bleed easily; oozing dampness of rectum; early and profuse menses, cervical erosion and easy bleeding, especially of aged; leukorrhea with bloody mucus; ecchymosis.

< open air; cold spirits
< injuries; **odor of coffee**
< climacteric; evenings
< excessive hot or cold

> hot drinks
> hands near head
> moderate temperatures
> lying on affected side

Consider:

Calcarea carb (3)—See post partum hemorrhage.

Calcarea sulph (3)

Erigeron (3)—See post partum hemorrhage.

Ferrum met (3)—See post partum hemorrhage.

Ficus—See post partum hemorrhage; good for any hemorrhage.

Mercurius cor (3)

Natrum mur (3)

Nux vomica (3)

Pulsatilla (3)—See post partum hemorrhage.

Sepia (3)—See post partum hemorrhage.

Sulphur (3)—See post partum hemorrhage.

Symptoms in Kent's Repertory **Page**

Rectum, Hemorrhage, stool, during.......................619
Urine, Bloody.......................................681
Expectoration, Bloody...............................813
Chest, Hemorrhage...................................833
Generalities, Hemorrhage............................1365
Generalities, Hemorrhage, blood does not coagulate ...1365
Generalities, Pulse, weak...........................1397

HEMORRHOIDS

Most everyone has been affected with **hemorrhoids** at one time or another, as it is a condition associated with sedentary life styles, overindulgence, chronic constipation, liver disease and childbirth. It is caused most often by straining during passage of a hard stool which tears the rectal mucosa or from bearing down during childbirth. It is almost never considered a medical emergency unless there is a complete prolapse and severe pain. Sufficient amounts of blood can be lost with chronic conditions, which can lead to anemia.

If caught early, hemorrhoids are easily and effectively treated with homeopathic medicines, often causing a complete reversal of the damage. If the condition has occurred for some time, homeopathic medicines offer relief from the pain and bleeding but are not able to reverse the tissue damage which is present. Other nonsurgical methods such as galvanic and infrared coagulation used in conjunction with homeopathy will alleviate the suffering.

Aesculus (3)

Aggravated. night; **blind**; **bluish**; **chronic**; **external**; internal; **large**; **pregnancy**; agg. standing; preventing stool; strangulated; **agg. walking**; warm weather ameliorates; **agg. from wiping**; sensation as if a lump in anus, glass is in rectum or ball of needles; large, purple/blue; rarely bleed; sharp, pulsating, sticking pains; throbs; feels as if a worm is coming out; pain after stool which shoots up rectum; anus raw, sore; prolapse with stool; **burning in anus with chills up and down back**; large, hard, dry, stool; chilly.

< AM, on waking
< after stool; lying; stooping
< urinating; walking
< motion; after eating
< standing

> **cool**, open air, bathing
> bleeding of piles; kneeling
> continued exertion

Aloe (3)

Aggravated. in morning, awakes them; agg. beer; chronic; congested; **external**; **large**; agg. during menses; after purgations; **strangulated**; protrude with urination; give if sulphur should have worked but didn't ;ill effects of sedentary habits; constant bearing down sensation in rectum; **sense of insecurity in rectum**; stool passes with little effort, unnoticed; rectum sore after stool; **mucus and pain in rectum after stool**; hemorrhoids protrude like grapes; sore and tender; **burning in anus**, rectum; pain from naval to rectum; **sense of pulsation in rectum** after eating or flatus.

< **heat**; damp, summer
< early AM; after dysentery
< stepping hard; evening
< after eating, drinking

> cold applications; cool open air

Arsenicum alb (3)

Aggravated. night; blind; bluish; congested; in drunkards; external; large; strangulated; suppressed; agg. walking; external warmth ameliorates; **burning**; excoriating with stool; micro fissures; protrude and become blue; painful, spasmodic protrusion of rectum; excoriated skin around anus; **small**, **offensive**, **dark stool with protrusion**; **restlessness**; **nightly aggravations**; **fear**, **fright**, **worry**; **thirsty**, **desires ice cold drinks or warm drinks**; **chilly**.

< cold, **drinks**, **food**, air
< midnight, after 2 AM
< vegetables; **drinking**
< eruptions, suppressed, undeveloped
< tobacco; **exertion**; lying on part
< wet weather; right side
< seashore

> hot, **applications**, **food**
> warm drinks; motion
> elevating head
> company, sweating

Collinsonia (3)

Aggravated. night; blind; **chronic**; external; agg. during menses; agg. pregnancy; constant bleeding; hemorrhoids with backache and **obstinate constipation**; piles bleeding or blind and protruding; may have **alternating constipation and diarrhea**; **sensation of sharp sticks in rectum**, **constriction**; aching in anus and hypogastrium; **itching of anus** (Rat, Teuc); dysentery with tenesmus; vascular engorgement of rectum; bleeding piles, alternating with heart, chest or rheumatic symptoms; anal prolapse.

< piles, during, suppressed
< night; pregnancy
< cold; excitement, sitting
< slightest mental emotion

> eating
> bleeding of piles

Hamamelis (3)

Bluish; **external**; **large**; **bleeding is intense with stool**; **bleeding with soreness**; anus feels raw, **sore**; pulsation in rectum; painless bleeding followed by prostration which is out of proportion to loss of blood; dark blood; milk leg, hemorrhoids, sore nipples after confinement; passive venous bleeding; pain goes along spermatic cord.

< injury; bruises; pressure
< air, open, humid, cold
< motion, touch, jarring
< warm moist air

Lachesis (3)

Bluish; chronic; **external**; hard; internal; large; agg. during menses; pregnancy during; preventing stool; protrude during stool; **strangulated**; ulcerating; inflamed with hammering pains; big, blue, purple piles; bleeds dark blood; pains shoot upward; sensation of a weight on left side; chronic constipation, < heat; **offensive stool**; anus **feels tight** as if nothing can go through; pains dart up rectum with cough, sneezing; constant urging in rectum, not for stool; pain from anus to navel; **left sided complaints**; **move to right**; **flushes of heat**, **loquacity**; thirsty but fears to drink; restless, uneasy; chilly.

< sleep, after, AM
< heat; sun, room, drinks
< swallowing, empty
< pressure of clothes
< slightest touch
< retarded discharges

> open air; free secretions
> hard pressure
> cold drinks; bathing part

< start & close of menses
< climaxis; **alcohol**
< cloudy weather
< left side; closing eyes

Muriatic acid (3)

Bluish; in children; congested; **external**; large; agg. motion; agg. parturition; protrude during stool; **agg. touch**; protrude during urination; **agg. walking**; **agg. from wiping**; very tender big, blue hemorrhoids; will not use toilet paper; piles like a bunch of grapes, burn when touched; involuntary stools while urinating; anal itching and prolapse with urination; **during pregnancy**; **bluish**, **hot**, **stitching**; sore piles > heat; **restlessness**, irritable, peevish; **loud moaning**; **suffers in silence**.

< touch; wet weather	> motion; warmth
< walking; cold drinks	> lying on left side
< bathing; sitting	
< human voice	
< before midnight	

Nitric acid (3)

Rectal bleeding at night; blind; chronic; external; **large**; protrude during stool; agg. by touch; ulcerating; protrude during urination; agg. walking; agg. by warm weather; very sharp pains; associated with fissures, cracks; watery, excoriating stool, feels like a knife; spasm of anus from pain; anus protrudes with stool; bright red blood; great straining with stool; little passes; violent cutting pains **after stools**, **lasts for hours** (Rat); hemorrhoids bleed easily; irritable, exhausted after stool; **splinter** like pains; dry, cracked skin; easy perspiration; hateful, profane; itching; eczematous anus or oozes moisture; **chilly**; thirsty.

< touch; **jarring**, slightest causes	> gliding motion; riding
< motion; noise; milk	> mild weather
< after eating; **cold**; air, dampness	> steady pressure
< night, evenings; weather changes	
< heat of bed; mental exertion	

Nux vomica (3)

Aggravated beer; **blind**; **chronic**; **congested**; **in drunkards**; excitement; external; **internal**; **large**; in pregnancy; strangulated; **suppressed**; agg. touch; **one big hemorrhoid**; hard stool, **ineffectual urging**; straining; may bleed continuously; itches at night; prolapse; constriction of rectum; **itching**; very painful; alternating constipation and diarrhea; desires stimulants; sensation as if more stool remains; flatus; **chilly**, thirsty; piles are > with cold; **constant uneasy feeling in rectum.**

< early AM; cold, open air	**> free discharges**
< drafts; **uncovering**	> naps; wrapping head
< sedentary; **coffee, stimulants**	> resting; hot drinks
< mental exertion; overeating	> milk; moist air
< vexation; fatigue; disturbed sleep	> evenings; strong pressure
< anger; noise; touch; **pressure** of clothes, especially around waist	

Paeonia (3)

Congested; external; prevents stool; **strangulated**; ulcerating; **agg. after wiping**; intense pain, similar to nitric acid but patient walks around; **lasts for 6 hours; spreads cheeks due to pains**; biting; **itching in anus**; burning after stool, then internal chilliness; painful ulcer, oozing offensive moisture on perineum; **hemorrhoids, fissures, ulceration of anus and perineum, purple, covered with crusts**; pains with and after stool.

< stool, touch	> hot soaks
< night; motion	

Phosphorus (3)

Internal; chronic; agg. during menses; protrude with stool; agg. touch; bright red blood, unclotted; long, narrow hard stools like a dogs; with blood; **great weakness after stool**; **white**, hard stools; **fetid stools and flatus**; desire for stool lying on left side; anus open, prolapsed; suddenness of symptoms; restless; involuntary stools; **thirst** for cold drinks; **chilly**.

< lying on left side; back	> in dark; cold food
< emotions; talking; touch	> lying on right side

< odors; light	> cold; open air
< cold; **hands**, open air	> sleep; rubbing
< warm ingesta; salt; puberty	> sitting up
< sexual excesses; weather changes	
< windy; cold; thunderstorms	
< AM, PM; mental fatigue	
< ascending stairs	

Pulsatilla (3)

Aggravated. night; blind hemorrhoids; congested; external; **internal**; large; before and during menses; agg. parturition; agg. from wiping; itching and sticking pains; **no two stools alike**; venous congestion, varicose veins; green mucus in stools; **desires open air**; **thirstless**, **changeable**; **peevish**; **chilly**; very sensitive.

< warmth, **air**, **room**, clothes	**> cold**; **fresh open air**
< getting feet wet; **beginning motion**	> uncovering; gentle motion
< suppressions; **evening**; **rest**	**> erect posture**
< lying; one side	> weeping
< rich foods; **fats**, ices, eggs	> cold applications
< puberty; **pregnancy**	
< before menses	
< towards evening	
< allowing feet to hang down	

Ratanhia (2)

External; **protrude during stool**; **agg. touch**; hemorrhoids; **fissures**; abscesses; **severe burning and deep cutting pain** during stool, for hours; intense **burning**; protrusion with hard stool; rectum aches as if full of broken glass; anus feels constricted; dry heat at anus with sudden knife like stitches; stools forced with great effort; oozing; itching of anus; **pinworms**; hemorrhoids > cold water; thirsty; anxiety about health (Ars); **very sympathetic** (Phos).

< night; anxiety; heat	> cool bathing
< exertion	> walking in open air
< touch	> movement
< after stool	

Sepia (3)

External; internal; hard; large; **agg. by milk**; agg. parturition; during pregnancy; agg. touch; agg. walking; chronic constipation and congestion; **sense of lump in rectum**; little balls form; prolapse; **pain shoots upward**; bleeding at stool; cannot strain; great tenesmus; stool of dark brown round balls that stick together; soft stool difficult; **almost constant oozing from rectum**; sensation of relaxation, bearing down in abdomen; rectum constricted and powerless, no urging for days; stool, followed by gelatinous mucus; **feels cold**, even in a warm room; **averse** to family, sympathy; irritable, **very sad**; dreads being alone; weeps telling symptoms; thirstless; some thirst.

< cold, **air**, north wind	**> violent motion**
< wet; snowy	> warmth, cold drinks
< sexual excesses; before menses	> pressure; drawing limbs up
< pregnancy; abortion	> cold bathing; after sleep
< AM and evenings	
< after first sleep; left side	
< before thunderstorms	

Sulphur (3)

Aggravated night; **agg. beer**; bluish; **chronic**; congested; **external and internal**; **large**; agg. during menses, suppressed menses; agg. parturition; pregnancy; agg. standing; strangulated; **suppressed**; **agg. touch**; **agg. from walking**; agg. wiping; **several small hemorrhoids**; itching, pruritus ani; awakes at night with itching; protrude with straining, may get prolapse; congested, bleeds occasionally (dark blood); fissures, fistula develops; sharp pain shoots upward with stool; sore, painful, bruised, pulsating anus; **redness around anus**; child afraid due to pain; > with spicy food, alcohol; **early AM diarrhea**; chilly, **thirsty**; can be thirstless.

< suppressions; **bathing**; milk	> open air; motion
< heated, **exertion**, **bed**	> warm applications
< atmospheric changes; speaking	> sweating; dry heat
< 11 AM; full moon; climacteric	> lying on right side
< rest, standing; night	> drawing up affected limbs

Consider:

Ammonium carb (2)

Protrusion after stool with long lasting pains; cannot walk; protrude independent of stool; burning and itching in anus prevents sleep; **< menses**; **bleeding piles**; piles > lying down.

Carbo veg (3)

Protruding **blue** piles; suppurating; offensive; swelling; burning in rectum; oozing of fluid; flatulence; **acrid**, **corrosive moisture from rectum**; white hemorrhoids, **pains after stool**; anus excoriated.

Causticum (3)

Intolerably painful piles **< walking**; **large**; **agg**. **touch**; fissures of anus; small, hard, tough stools; rectum sore and burns.

Graphites (3)

Burning piles; smarting; sore, itching anus; fissures, varices of anus; large, difficult, knotty stools; **agg**. **by wiping**; dryness, cracks in skin.

Kali carb (3)

Painful, **burn like fire**, copious bleeding; much distension and swelling inside; anal fistula; burning temporarily > with cold water, cold applications; **congested**; **large**; **agg**. **parturition**; pain with cough; easy prolapse; sharp, stitching pains; may be constipated but with a soft stool.

Teucrium

Itching of anus; **constant irritation and itching**, **especially in bed**, **from Ascaris**; **nightly restlessness**; crawling sensation in the rectum after stool; polyps of rectum, and/or nose.

Symptoms in Kent's Repertory	**Page**
Rectum, Constipation, pregnancy during	608
Rectum, Constipation, sedentary habits	608
Rectum, Fissure/Fistula	617
Rectum, Bleeding, stool during	619

INFLUENZA

Influenza or the **"flu"** is a common occurrence worldwide. It is often seasonal in nature, occurring mostly in the fall and winter. Influenza epidemics can be followed from one part of the country to another and will vary in severity depending upon the strain of virus. Each year the virus changes slightly as it adapts to its human hosts. Therefore, flu vaccines are often ineffective as they are no longer similar to the current virus.

Homeopathic medicines administered at the onset of symptoms will abate the condition altogether or shorten its course. Clinical experience suggests that administration of the nosode **Influenzinum** prior to the flu season acts as a prophylactic to prevent the disease. Certainly, coupled with preventive measures and periods of rest during infection, homeopathic medicines are highly effective in influenza.

Influenza becomes a problem for the very young or the elderly as their tolerance ranges are narrower, and they cannot respond as well to treatment. If the condition continues to persist for longer than its normal course of between 3 to 14 days, or if it evolves into other conditions, medical attention should be sought.

Baptisia

Rapid onset, prostration, stupidity, mottled face, bleeding and putrid mouth; patient looks drunk; is confused, delirious; dissociated; **feels there are two of him**; limbs are scattered, restless and tosses and turns; **septic conditions**; **great muscle soreness & putrid phenomena are always present**; offensive secretions; epidemic influenza; inability to think, confusion; pressure at root of nose; skin feels tight across forehead, head feels too large, **heavy**, **numb**; eyeballs are sore, brain feels sore; **besotted look**; dark red face; **can swallow liquids only** as solid food gags; heavy, drowsy with flushed face and wandering mind.

< humid heat; fog; indoors
< pressure; on awaking; cold wind
< thinking about pains

Bryonia

Sleep, heavy, lethargic with flushed face, contused face; dislikes being disturbed; thick coated tongue, **thirsty for large drinks of cold water**; backache, headache, eye ache, limbs ache; **dryness of mucous membranes**; **stitching**, **tearing pains**; **weakness**; children do not want to be carried; **very irritable**; determined; wants to be left alone, go home; head—**bursting**, **splitting headache**; **< motion**, sensation as if everything is pressing out, becomes seated in occiput; frontal headache; nose—**frequent bleeding of nose**, **when menses should appear**; coryza with aching forehead; eyes—pressing pain; sore to touch and movement; pain behind eyes; mouth—**dry**, **parched lips**, **cracked**; **dryness with excessive thirst**; tongue coated yellowish, dark brown; throat—dry; touch, thick mucus; respiratory—soreness, hoarseness; dry cough at night; **must sit up**; **< after eating or drinking**; **stitches in chest**; **< coming into warm rooms**; extremities—knees stiff, painful; **joints swollen**, **hot**; **pulse is full**, **hard**, **quick**, **tense**; chill with external coldness, internal heat; sour sweat after slight exertion; feels "under the weather" prior to onset; **averse to least motion**; **dry very hard stools**.

< motion; **deep breathing**
< dry heat, cold, **stooping**
< becoming hot, **hot room**
< taking cold
< eating; **vexation**; touch
< early AM; suppressions
< vegetables

> pressure; rest
> lying on painful part
> cool open air
> quiet
> cloudy, damp days
> drawing knees up
> heat to inflamed part

Eupatorium perf

Warm, mild weather flu's; **extreme aching deep in bones**; back and legs feeling as if bones will break; restlessness; bed is uncomfortable, feels hard; increased heat and no perspiration; weakness; head—throbbing pain, **soreness of eyeballs**; **occipital pain after lying down with sense of weight**; respiratory—coryza with sneezing; **hoarseness and cough with soreness of chest**; **chronic** loose cough

< night; cough relieved by getting on hands and knees; must hold chest (Bry); extremities—**aching pain in back** and muscles; **soreness of skin**; **aching in arms and wrists**; perspiration relieves all symptoms except headache; chill between 7–9 AM **preceded by thirst and aching and soreness of bones**; knows chill is coming on because they can't drink enough; chill is < movement; tends to have chronic episodes; leukopenia often accompanies condition; **thirsty**.

< cold air; motion	> vomiting bile; sweating
< 7–9 AM; 3rd or 7th day	> lying on face
< lying on part; coughing	> conversation
< smell or sight of food (Colch)	> getting on hands and knees

Gelsemium

Warm, mild winter flu's or summer; associated with nervous shock, fear, fright, emotional upset; much exhaustion, weariness, prostration; **dizzy**, **dull**, **droopy**, **drowsy**; cannot exert himself to move or turn; wants to be left alone; face is suffused and congested; thirstless; **trembling**, **muscle weakness** cold and damp brings on complaints; **apathetic about their illness**; lack any fear; head—feels heavy; **band feeling** around head; dull ache with heaviness of eyelids; feel bruised; **pain in temple to ear**; > with head held high; eyes—can hardly open eyes; blurred vision; **orbital neuralgia with contraction and twitching of muscles**; one pupil dilated the other contracted; nose—sneezing; dryness of fossae; watery excoriating discharge; coryza with dull headache and fever; face—**hot**, **heavy**, **besotted look**, **flushed**; neuralgia; chin quivers; lower jaw dropped; mouth—putrid taste and breath, numb, thick yellowish coated, **trembling** tongue; difficulty swallowing especially warm food; pains in neck; respiration—slowness of breath; prostration; dry cough with sore chest and fluent coryza; aphonia; **no thirst**; copious profuse, clear urine which makes things >; **vertigo**; **dread** of falling; **wants to be held** due to shaking; chills run up and down back.

< emotions; **dread**; surprise	> profuse urination
< shock; motion	> perspiration; shaking
< spring, **humid**, foggy, muggy weather	> alcoholic drinks; open air
	> mental effort
< heat of summer; periodically	> bending forward

< tobacco; dentition; gas
< thinking of ailments; at 10 AM
> continued motion

Nux vomica

Past exposure to cold East or NE wind; patient feels cold, shivers from motion; moving bed clothes brings on shivers; is disagreeable, ill tempered, snappy, wants to be left alone; aching in all limbs; **irritable**, **sensitive to noise**, **odors**; does not want to be touched; **cannot sleep after 3 AM until towards morning**, **> after a nap**; head—sensitive scalp; headache over eyes; desires to press hard against something; **headache in sun** (Glon, Nat c); feels distended; sore; eyes—photophobia, < in AM; orbital neuralgia with watering of eyes; dry sensation of inner canthi; twitching of eyes; nose—**stuffed up especially at night**; occurs after exposure to cold, dry, < in warm rooms; fluent coryza during day; stuffed nose alternates between nostrils; acrid discharge and still feels stuffed; throat—**rough**, **scraped feeling**; **tickling sensation** in AM; constricted pharynx, swollen uvula; tightness and tension feeling; pain **stitches to ear**; respiration—hoarseness from catarrh with **scraping in throat**, **asthma with fullness in stomach in AM or after eating**; **cough brings on bursting headache**, feels as if it has torn something loose in chest; **oppressed breathing**; dry cough, may have bloody expectoration; extremities—arms and hands go to sleep; sensation of a sudden loss of power in AM; **must sit up to turn over in bed**; **body is burning hot**, **especially face**, **yet cannot move or uncover without feeling chill**; sour perspiration; **may not allow himself to be covered even though chilled with uncovering**; **violent vomiting**; **chilly**.

< early AM; **uncovering**
< cold, **open air**, drafts
< coffee; stimulants
< overeating; sedentary habits
< mental exertion; disturbed sleep
< anger, noise, odors, touch; light
< pressure, of clothes

> free discharges
> naps
> wrapping head; hot drinks
> milk; moist air
> strong pressure
> damp, wet weather

Rhus tox

After exposure to wet, damp; aching in all limbs < on beginning to move; **much restlessness**, **has to keep moving**; **cloudy sen-**

sorium; tongue—coated with a red tip, dry and red at edges. Head—vertigo with rising, **heavy**, brain feels loose; headache in occiput, goes from frontal to occiput, painful to touch, sensitive scalp; eyes—swollen, red; photophobia; painful with turning or pressure; circumscribed corneal infection; nose—sneezing, tip of nose red; swelling, sore; face—facial neuralgia with chilliness, < evenings; **swollen face**, erysipelas; cheek bones sensitive to touch; throat—**swollen glands**, sore; sticking pains with swallowing; respiratory—dry, tickling sensation behind sternum; cough from midnight to morning, **during chill or with putting hands out of bed**; chilly, as if cold water poured over him, followed by heat; **does not tolerate cold fresh air, makes the skin painful**; **stiffness of limbs**, sore joints, wants to stretch limbs; aching in all bones (Eup per); tearing pains; dreams of great exertion, sleepless before midnight; **thirsty**, **chilly**.

< during sleep; cold, wet weather	> warm; dry; motion
< after rain; night; during rest	> change of position; rubbing
	> stretching

Consider:

Aconite

Chill after cold, dry wind exposure, affected within a few hours; hot burning face; **restlessness**, **fear**, **agonized**; faint feeling on sitting up.

Allium cepa

After exposure to cold damp wind; **bland watery discharge from eyes, excoriating discharge from nose**; throat and larynx raw, extending to chest; tickling cough and tearing pain; left sided nasal catarrh.

Arsenicum alb

Restlessness, prostration, weakness, pain, headache, **much thirst for sips of warm drinks**; < after midnight.

Causticum

Comes on with cold, dry East wind; neuralgic pain, face aches; hollow cough producing escape of urine (Puls); sip of cold water relieves cough; limbs feel as if beaten; chilliness during temperature leading to perspiration with no heat; dark redness of tonsils and soft palate; bitter taste, **constriction**, **contraction of esophagus**, **painful sore throat**; constant desire for water; no appetite; lumps feel compressed; difficult breathing; fears going to sleep due to nightmares and **sense of suffocation**; neck feels tired; stiffness, pain, aching and drawing in arms and legs; **sore and bruised** feeling; chill with rheumatic pains and soreness all over; chill 11 AM; **adynamic fevers**; air hunger > standing.

Hepar sulph

Cold, dry windy weather; North and NE winds; feels cold in back of neck with moving; sticking pain in throat; **very sensitive to pain**; irritable, nasty; covers back of neck, even in bed; much perspiration.

Influenzinum

For patients who trace their chronic problems back to a case of the flu; deafness coming on slowly and is progressive, after flu.

Oscillococcinum

Best to give at the first onset of a flu; anxiety, pale, shivering, fixed obsessional ideas; obstinacy; washes hands often; fears storms; oculo-nasal discharge; nasal obstruction and sneezing; serous to mucopurulent discharge; pain in frontal sinuses; dry irritating cough; piercing pain both ears with decreased hearing.

Phosphoric acid

Apathy, **debility**; highly emotional; grief causes debility; **emaciated**, **tired** and speaks in a monotone; **averse to mental effort** due to it being tiring; dark circles around the eyes, sunken face, pale; spaciness due to inability to think; **< from loss of vital fluids**, sexual excesses; **painless diarrhea with exhaustion** but is **> from diarrhea**; **milky urinary sediment**; **is thirsty** (Gels opp.).

Pulsatilla

Flu from getting wet, wet feet; shivers up and down back with increased temperature; feeling of cold water pouring down back;

much catarrh with congestion in back of nose and throat; > warm stuffy room, > open air; thirstless; < evenings.

Pyrogen

Similar to Eupatorium; has to move even though it hurts; bed uncomfortable and hard; much perspiration, bed is soaked; delirious and feels he has too many parts to his body; **sepsis**, pulse decreased and temperature increased or vice versa; pulse abnormally rapid, **out of proportion to temperature**; chill begins in back; **sweating does not cause a drop in temperature**; tongue is red and dry, foul breath; **discharges are very offensive**; painless throbbing of head; anxiety, loquacious, **restless**, think they are in a dream; throbbing in vessels of neck; numbness of hands, arms, feet; profuse hot sweat; **feels bruised**; **sore**, **chilly**.

< cold damp	> heat; hot bath; pressure
< motion	> motion

Scutellaria

Consider as a post influenza or viral fatigue remedy; inability to study or concentrate (Ph ac), with stupor or **dull headache**; **sense of confusion**, being off balance, vertigo; reality is askew; problems with depth perception which may follow ringing in the ears; low level of anxiety; sensitive to noise (Nux v); sleeplessness, restless (Ars); confused articulation of words (Thuja); nausea, gas and abdominal distention with out modalities; headache is < with activity or excitement; chilly or are sensitive to heat.

Symptoms in Kent's Repertory	**Page**
Head, Pain, catarrhal	137
Head, Pain, coryza, with.	138
Head, Sensitiveness of brain	229
Eye, Falling of lids	240
Eye, Heat in	241
Eye, Inflammation, catarrhal cold.	242
Eye, Lachrymation, coryza during	245
Eye, Pain, aching	251

STINGS OF INSECTS

Insect bites and **stings** more commonly occur in the spring, summer and early fall due to the larger number of insects which are present. In warmer climates and in buildings during the winter months, insect bites may occur, especially those of spiders. In most cases the person will experience faintness, weakness and mild nausea, while the area bitten becomes red, painful and swollen. This condition usually abates in a few days.

If the **bite becomes infected**, a red streak may begin to travel from the site as the infection spreads through the lymphatics. This is the beginning of blood poisoning, and if not responding to homeopathic treatment, the person needs to be seen by a physician.

In some cases, the lesion will begin to break down after a few days due to the poisons which have been left in the skin. **Necrotic skin** is a breeding ground for bacteria which will lead to sepsis if left unchecked. This is always accompanied by a fever.

In some cases, the person may react immediately to the insect bite by going into **anaphylactic shock**. This is a life-threatening condition which requires emergency treatment.

Apis (2)

Stinging pains; **swollen**, **sensitive** and **sore** skin after a bite, with **rapid swelling** of part or whole body; intolerable itching, especially at night; stinging and burning pains (Anthr, Ars), pains of carbuncles, abscesses, boils; body covered with large, elevated white wheals; scarlet eruptions; nettle-like rash; dry, hot skin, may alternate with perspiration; edematous swellings; patient is **> with cold applications**, **< with heat**; will feel fatigued, apathetic and drowsy; poor concentrating ability.

< heat, warm room	**> cold, applications**
< touch	> open air

Belladonna (2)

Rapid and **violent swelling** with **heat sensation** and scarlet redness; cutting, sharp, knife-like pains; rapid spreading of redness and swelling; **alternating redness and paleness** of the skin; shining of skin; skin is smooth, tight, shining and is < touch (if vesicles are present, consider Rhus t); dry, hot burning of skin, **which burns the examiner's hand as if touching a hot stove**; may have a small, rapid pulse with difficult respiration; **no thirst**, **anxiety or fear**.

< touch; jarring

Caladium (2)

Burning and **itching sensation** in small areas of the skin with insect bites; inclination to touch burning parts but not scratch them; skin feels rough, dry; may have skin rash which alternates with asthma; **fatigue diminishes with the appearance of the eruptions**; (may have modalities similar to Ars, Bry).

< motion

> cool air
> perspiration

Cedron (2)

Reported to counter act the effects of snake and insect bites in the tincture to 3x potency.

Lachesis (2)

Hot, **bluish-purple** swellings or **blue-black** swellings (Anthr), with much prostration; tendency to ulceration, inflammation, bleeding and spreading wounds; bluish color surrounding wounds; **very sensitive to touch**, **warmth** and pressure of dressings (Bell, Bry); patient may be very agitated, loquacious, laughing, angry or in a rage; mental symptoms get better with discharge of the lesion; patient is **< heat** but may also be aggravated by cold; chilly.

< extremes of temperature
< heat, **touch**, **pressure**

> discharges

Ledum (3)

Antidotal to insect stings, poison oak; **good for any puncture wound**, especially if **part is cold**; tetany or twitching of muscles near the wound; edema from wounds; ***coldness of affected part but patient does not want part covered or warm*** and is **> with cold applications** (Secale); may have hot, hard swelling with tearing pains; ecchymosis which remains long after pain and inflammation has left (follows Arnica well); thirsty; **chilly**.

< warmth	> cold applications
< movement	> rest

Natrum mur (2)

Itching and prickling of the skin; rash with stinging sensation, may cover whole body; nettle—like rash after exercise, < exertion; shooting pains; thought to antidote effects of insect bites, stings.

< heat	> open air

Urtica urens (3)

Itching of skin with red, raised blotches, swellings; **prickly heat**, erythema with burning and stinging, **> *warmth*** (opp Apis); numbness and smarting of the skin with swelling; **first-degree burns, scalds** (topically or internally); may have rheumatic symptoms which alternate with nettle rash; **antidotes shellfish poisoning**.

< after sleep	**> warmth**
< cold, cool	
< touch	

Symptoms in Kent's Repertory **Page**

Face, Bloated 353
Mouth, Swelling, tongue after stings of insects 421
Skin, Stinging 1331
Skin, Stings, of insects 1331
Skin, Swelling, hard/spongy/stinging 1332

LARYNGITIS

A condition caused by an **inflammation** of the **larynx** or "voice box" which results in a loss of the person's ability to talk except in a whisper. There may be a number of causes of the inflammation such as overuse, straining the vocal cords, or infection of the throat and larynx.

Other causes which must be considered but are less likely are a tumor on the vocal cords, a disruption of the nerve which leads to the larynx, or possibly a stroke affecting the speech center of the brain.

As with any other medical condition, if the person does not respond to treatment, a medical evaluation is in order.

Aconite (2)

Inflammation of **larynx**, trachea; exposure to dry, cold air; **high fever**; chills; hot, dry skin; no perspiration; **restlessness**, **fear**, **anxiety**, fear of death, sensitive to cold air on chest; difficult inspiration; husky voice; throat feels raw; larynx sensitive; dry, short, hacking cough **< night**, **after midnight**; sudden onset; **hoarse voice**; loss of voice from fright; from overuse; **thirst**, larynx sensitive to touch; wants to cough but cannot.

< fright, **shock**, vexation
< cold wind, dry wind
< sleeping in sun; touch
< noise; light; dentition; menses
< night; lying on side
< warm room; tobacco smoke

> open air; lying
> warm sweat

Antimonium crud (3)

Inflammation of larynx, **in singers**; from becoming heated; from motion; roughness of voice from overuse; scarcely able to utter a word; < from becoming overheated, < from rest; violent spasms in larynx, as if throat filled with a plug; cough < from becoming heated; **voice harsh**, **badly pitched**; no thirst; **thick coated white tongue**; chilly; great heat in throat while moving in open air.

< **cold**, **bathing**, damp, **water**	> open air; rest
< **overeating**; acids; sweets	> moist warmth
< **heat**, **summer** sun, overheating	
< evenings; wet poultices	

Argentum nit (3)

Chronic laryngitis of singers' inflammation of larynx; **sensation of a splinter in throat on swallowing**; **strangulated sensation**; **high notes cause cough**; continued and vain efforts to swallow; pain and soreness with swallowing food; dry, spasmodic cough; dark red appearance of throat; fauces; fearful; **nervous**; **impulsive**, < in crowds; intolerance of heat; **strong desire for sweets**; pains increase and decrease gradually; chilly; **thirsty**.

< **anxiety**; suspense	> **cool air**, bath
< in room; **sweets**	> hard pressure; motion
< lying on right side; looking down	
< drinking; crowds	> eructations
< warmth; night	
< cold food; **left side**; menses	

Bromium (3)

Inflammation of larynx, **from becoming heated**; inflammation of trachea; throat feels raw; tickling in trachea with inspiration; **dry cough with hoarseness**, burning behind sternum; little expectoration; voice weak, soft; cannot speak clearly; laryngeal constriction which is painful to the touch; danger of **suffocation from accumulation of mucus**; deep hoarseness < if heated; chilly; some thirst.

< **warm**, **damp**, overheating	> nosebleeds
< chilled while hot	> at sea; motion
< sea bathing; until midnight	
< dust; drafts; warm room	
< lying on left side	

Carbo veg (3)

Inflammation of the larynx, trachea; loss of voice **evening**; night, cold air; **on exertion**; chronic laryngitis in the elderly; deep, rough voice; failing on slightest exertion; **cough, with burning in the chest**; painless hoarseness, < cold weather; ulcerative pain in larynx, putrid sputum; hyperemia of mucous membranes of larynx; **has never recovered since previous illness**; **weakness**, **icy coldness**; **dusky face**; wants to be fanned, thirst for cold water; thirsty, chilly.

< warmth; **depletions**	**> eructations**; cool air
< **exhausting diseases**	> elevating feet
< old age; **high living**; rich food	**> from being fanned**
< over-lifting; walking in open air	> cold
< extreme temperatures; humid	
< wind on head; cooling off	

Causticum (3)

Inflammation of larynx; loss of voice from exposure to cold, **from paralysis**; from overuse, **singers**, **sudden loss**; own voice roars in ears; raw throat, larynx; dry cough, hurts and makes chest sore; difficult expectoration; **chronic hoarseness after acute laryngitis**; **paralysis after surgery**; laryngeal muscles refuse to act; loss of voice from anger; **intensely sympathetic**, sad, hopeless, ailments from long-lasting grief, sudden emotions.

< air, **cold**, **dry**, **wind**	**> cold drinks**; washing
< temperature extremes; stooping	> warmth of bed
< 3–4 AM; **or evening**; coffee	> gentle motion
< exertion; weather changes	> damp, wet weather

Kali bic (2)

Inflammation of larynx; in damp weather; inflammation of trachea; tickling in larynx; **profuse**, **yellow**, **thick**, **gelatinous**, **sticky mucus** in throat, chronic laryngitis with congestion; coughs and gags; pseudomembranous deposits on tonsils, soft palate, which can extend to bronchi; fissured pharynx; burning of pharynx extending to stomach; asthma 2–3 AM; thirsty; **chilly**.

< cold, damp, air, spring	> heat; motion
< undressing	
< morning; 2–3 AM; after sleep	
< protruding tongue	
< hot weather; alcohol; beer	
< suppressed catarrh	

Phosphorus (3)

Inflammation of larynx, gangrenous; loss of voice from prolonged talking; dryness of pharynx, fauces; **larynx very painful**; clergyman's sore throat; violent tickling in pharynx while speaking; **cannot talk due to pain in larynx**; < evenings, 8 PM–12 midnight; weak voice; hoarse, gruff; chilliness with cough; **craves cold drinks**; low spirits, easily vexed; dread to be alone; oversensitive; **chilly**; **thirsty**.

< lying on left side; **back**	> eating; sleep
< emotions; talking; touch; odors	> cold food; water to face
< light; morning, evenings	> rubbing; sitting up
< mental fatigue; salt	> in dark; open air
< weather changes; thunderstorms	
< warm food; **cold hands**, open air	

Consider:

Apis

Edema, short of breath; laryngeal spasms; < lying down, heat, hot drinks; > if cough, **cold**; consider if Belladonna fails.

Arum triphyllum (2)

Acute laryngitis; voice is hoarse, weak then gives out; voice cracks; cannot control it; goes to a high pitch; changes pitch; feels sore; roar in throat; swollen sensation due to mucus and constant pain.

Belladonna (2)

Sudden onset; larynx dry, hot; pain with swallowing; bright red vocal cords; feeble voice; averse to drinks; constricted feeling in throat; **dilated pupils**.

Calcarea carb

Chronic laryngitis; cough, primarily at night; very hoarse and irritated larynx; small amounts of frothy mucus.

Sambucus

Laryngeal spasm, epiglottitis; springs out of bed choking; gasps for breath.

Sanguinaria (2)

Acute edema of larynx; feels swollen; epiglottitis; **dry with thick mucus**; has to sit up to cough; < lying down; red discoloration to cheeks with cough.

Spongia (2)

First stages, **dry**, irritating cough as if sponging throat, **burning**, < night; **tickling in throat**; **sensitive to touch**, **< touch**; **> after eating**.

Symptoms in Kent's Repertory	**Page**
External Throat, Clothing agg.	471
Larynx & Trachea, Inflammation, singers in/speakers	749
Larynx & Trachea, Pain, larynx, talking while	752
Larynx & Trachea, Paralysis, larynx	755
Larynx & Trachea, Voice, hoarseness	759
Larynx & Trachea, Voice, overuse of/singing from	760
Larynx & Trachea, Voice, lost, paralysis/singers/sudden	761

NAUSEA AND VOMITING OF PREGNANCY

Early morning **nausea and vomiting associated with pregnancy** is a fairly common occurrence in the first few months following conception. It is felt to be a sign of a healthy pregnancy, but its absence does not mean that there is a problem with the fetus or pregnancy. The amount of nausea and/or vomiting present may also vary from one pregnancy to another with the same person.

The condition can become serious if there is violent, ineffectual retching or if accompanied by loss of large amounts of gastric secretions resulting in loss of electrolytes and hydrochloric acid. Prolonged occurrence of nausea and vomiting may also indicate that there is a toxemic condition present which needs medical attention.

Arsenicum alb (2)

Diarrhea and vomiting; vomiting comes on immediately especially if cold; from alcohol use, **food poisoning**; clutches abdomen, rolls on ground; unable to drink wine; **burning sensation** in abdomen; **cannot bear the sight or smell of food** (Colch, Sep); **drinks much but a little at a time**; anxiety in pit of stomach; craves acids, coffee; eructations excoriate the pharynx; long-lasting eructations; vomits blood, bile, green mucus or brown-black mixed with blood; stomach is raw, irritable; dyspepsia from vinegar, acids, ice cream, ice water, tobacco; everything swallowed seems to lodge in esophagus; craves milk; **ill effects of vegetable diet**; **melon**, **watery fruits**; **great thirst**; **restless**, **anxious**, **chilly**.

< cold, **ice**, **drinks**, **food**,	**> hot applications**, **food**,
< cold air	> warm drinks
< after midnight; 2 AM	> motion; sitting erect
< vegetables, **drinking**	**> elevating head**
< exertion; tobacco	> company; sweating

< suppressed eruptions
< wet weather; seashore
< right side

Asarum (3)

Loss of appetite; flatulence, eructations; vomiting; **desires alcoholic drinks**; tobacco tastes bitter; nausea < after eating; clean tongue; great faintness; **undigested stool**; **always feels cold**; **excessive nervous sensibility**; scratching on silk, paper is unbearable; violent vomiting; cold saliva; chilly.

< odors, cold	> washing
< motion	> damp, wet weather
< cold, dry weather	

Bryonia (2)

Nausea and faintness with rising up; abnormal hunger, loss of taste; **thirst for large quantities**; vomits bile and water immediately after eating; **stomach is sensitive to touch**; **pressure in stomach as if a stone after eating**; **irritable**; **averse to least motion**; nausea < on right side; heavy-load sensation in stomach; dry mouth, mucous membranes.

< motion, **stooping**, **exertion**	**> pressure**, **lying on painful side**
< dry heat, cold	**> cool**, **open air**; **quiet**
< becoming hot, **hot room**,	> cloudy, damp days
< hot weather	
< eating, **vexation**; talking	> drawing knees up
< vegetables; acids; touch	> heat to inflamed part
< taking cold; suppressions	> rest
< early AM; touch	

Cocculus

Motion sickness; **averse to food**; nausea with faintness and **vomiting**; **metallic taste**; paralysis of muscles of deglutition; dryness of esophagus; cramp in stomach during and after a meal; loss of appetite; desire for cold drinks, especially beer; smell of food disgusts (Colch); sensation in stomach as if one had been a long time without food until hunger gone; **profound sadness**; speaks hastily; slowness of mentation; thirsty, chilly; **empty, hollow feeling**; sensitive to cold; vertigo.

< motion; noise; touch
< loss of sleep; exertion; pain
< emotions; cold; open air
< eating; swimming; afternoon

Colchicum (2)

Severe nausea **from sight, smell** (especially fish), **or thought of food** (Ars sight, smell; Cocc smell, Sep); distention of abdomen with gas; not > with passing of gas; dry mouth, tongue; burns; gum and teeth pain; **thirsty**; pain in stomach; flatulence; **craves various things** but is averse to them when smelling them, nausea; burning or **icy coldness** of stomach; thirst for effervescent, alcoholic drinks; **cold and weak but sensitive and restless**; **acuteness of smell**.

< motion; touch; night	> warmth; rest
< vibration; loss of sleep	> doubling up; sitting
< cold weather, damp	> stooping
< weather changes	
< slight exertion; checked sweat	
< sundown to sunrise; stretching	
< mental exertion; smell of eggs, meat	

Ipecac (2)

Vomiting does not ameliorate condition; blood in vomitus; severe vomiting; profuse salivation; tries to vomit but does not make it better; **tongue usually clean**; **constant nausea** and vomiting; face is pale, twitches; vomits food, bile, blood, mucus; stomach feels relaxed as if hanging down; **no thirst**; repugnance to food; chilly; irritable.

< warmth; damp room	> open air
< overeating, ices, pork, rich food	
< periodically; warm wind	
< heat and cold	
< lying down; movement	

Kreosotum (3)

Nausea; vomiting of food several hours after eating; of sweetish water in AM; coldness feeling as if ice water in stomach; soreness > eating; bitter taste after swallowing water; frothy eructations; pressure in abdomen causes person to loosen clothing; acidity of vomitus excoriates mucosa of mouth; vomiting, especially from malignant disease of the stomach; chilly.

< dentition; pregnancy	> warmth; hot food; motion
< rest; cold; eating	
< lying; summer	
< 6 PM to 6 AM	
< open air	

Nux vomica (3)

Immediate vomiting, but will not come; much belching; sour taste; bitter, acid-tasting vomitus; **nausea in AM**, **after eating**; **weight and pain in stomach**; **< eating**; flatulence and **pyrosis (heartburn)**; **nausea and vomiting** with much retching; ravenous hunger, especially about a day before the attack; **region of stomach very sensitive to pressure** (Ars, Bry), feels bloated; pressure as if a stone **several hours after eating**; desires stimulants; loves fats; dyspepsia from strong coffee; **violent vomiting**; clothes feel oppressive around abdomen; thirsty; **chilly**.

< early AM; **cold**, **open air**	**> free discharges**
< uncovering; **coffee**	> naps; wrapping head
< sedentary habits; overeating	> resting; hot drinks
< mental exertion; fatigue, vexation	> milk; moist air
< disturbed sleep; stimulants	> evenings; strong pressure
< slightest causes, anger, noise, touch	
< pressure of clothes	
< dry, cold weather; odor of tobacco	

Phosphorus (2)

Vomits dark blood; chronic vomiting; good for vomiting post-anesthesia; sour taste and eructations after eating; **throws up mouthfuls of ingestion**; **water is vomited as soon as it gets warm in stomach**; cardiac opening seems contracted, too narrow; food vomited soon after swallowing (Alum, Bry) stomach pain > with cold food, drinks; **ill effects of eating too much salt**; **weak**, **empty**, **gone feeling in abdomen**; **craves cold drinks**; waterbrash; burning in stomach; **chilly**.

< lying on left side, **back**, painful side
< emotions; talking, touch, odors
< light; twilight
< cold, **hands**, open air
< warm food; **salt**
< sexual excesses
< weather changes, windy, cold
< thunderstorms; AM & PM
< mental fatigue

> eating; sleep
> cold, food, water to face
> rubbing; sitting up
> in dark
> lying on right side

Sepia (3)

Severe nausea; loathes food, **especially in AM**; empty, **gone feeling** with nausea; **gone feeling not > with eating** (Carb an); nausea at sight or smell of food (Ars, Colch); nausea < lying on side; band of pains around hypochondria; disposition to vomit after eating; burning in pit of stomach; longing for **vinegar**; acids, pickles; acid dyspepsia with bloating, sour eructations; loathes fat (Puls); **faint sinking at epigastrium**; gnawing hunger; **indifference** to loved ones; **irritable**, **sad**; dreads to be alone; weeps with telling symptoms; chilly.

< cold, air, wind; snowy
< sexual excesses; pregnancy
< abortion; AM & PM
< after first sleep
< washing; left side
< before a thunderstorm

> violent motion; warmth
> cold drinks; after sleep
> pressure; drawing limbs up
> cold bathing

Tabacum (3)

Face becomes pale; **seasickness**, cold sweat with nausea; skin turns pale green; ***incessant nausea*** < tobacco smoke (Phos); vomiting from least motion; **vomiting during pregnancy with much spitting**; **terrible faint**, **sinking feeling in pit of stomach**; sense of relaxation of stomach, with nausea (Ipecac); wants abdomen uncovered; heaviness in abdomen; **very despondent**, forgetful, discontent.

< motion; lying on left side	> cold; fresh air
< opening eyes	> twilight
< evening	> uncovering abdomen
< extremes of heat and cold	

Symptoms in Kent's Repertory	**Page**
Nose, Smell, sensitive to cooking food/food/strong odors	349
Stomach, Appetite, wanting food, at sight of	479
Stomach, Aversion, see specific food	480
Stomach, Heartburn, pregnancy, during	500
Stomach, Nausea, food, looking at/thought of	507
Stomach, Nausea, pregnancy, during	509
Stomach, Retching, ineffectual	526
Stomach, Vomiting, pregnancy, during	534

OBSTETRICAL & GYNECOLOGICAL

This section is provided as a guide for the use of homeopathic medicines during **labor and delivery**. It is not meant to be complete, and anyone doing births should have extensive training in both the use of herbal medicine and drug therapy as well as homeopathy. There are several references at the end of this book which would benefit anyone wishing to use homeopathy in an obstetric practice. It has been mine as well as other practitioners' experience that homeopathic medicines work very well obstetric practice.

LABOR PAINS

Aconite

Great distress, restless with each pain; **fears** of not delivering fetus or will die, something will go wrong; **vulva, vagina and os are dry; tender and undilatable**; sudden, violent, acute, burning thirst; dry, hot skin; bounding pulse.

< violent emotions, fright, shock	> open air; repose
< chilled by cold, dry wind	> warm sweat
< pressure; touch	
< noise, light, lying on side	

Actea spicata

Pains are of a tearing, distressing character and not located properly to effect expulsion; rheumatic women; great nervous excitement with violent spasmodic pains.

< change of weather; slight exertion

< cold, night; touch

Arnica

Flushed face, hot head with rest of body cool with each pain; violent pains distract her; feels sore and bruised in any position; often changes position with feeble pains; bed feels hard.

< injuries, bruises, shock	> lying with head low
< jarring	> outstretched
< labor, overexertion	
< touch; motion	

Aurum mur

Pains make her desperate; wants to jump out window, dash herself down; congestion in heat; palpitations; weak but sensitive to pain; hopeless depression.

< emotions; depression	> cool, open air
< mental exertion	> cold bathing
< cold; night (sunset to sunrise)	> music, getting warm, walking

Belladonna

Pains come and go suddenly; spasms of os uteri which is hot, dry and tender; slow, tedious labor; os doesn't dilate in proportion to pain; **face red with injected eyes**; burning heat; jerks; twitching; spasms; may get a headache from being jarred; pupils dilated; restless.

< heat, PM	> light covering
< drafts on head	> bending backward
< light; noise; jarring	> bed rest
< touch; pressure; motion	
< company	

Borax

Pains darting upward, with violent and frequent eructations; fears a downward motion; very sensitive to any noise; nervous, anxious.

< downward motion	> 11 PM
< sudden noises	
< cold, wet, uncovering	

Camphor

Pains have ceased; skin is cold, dry, shrunken; does not like to be covered; restless; **icy cold, yet averse to being covered**; internal burning heat; heat or sweat.

< suppression	> with covers; sensitive to cold air
< cold drafts	> free discharges
< mental exertion	> sweat, thinking of sweating

Carbo veg

Weak pains or cease from great debility; varicose vulva, **loss of fluids: air hunger**, exhausted; icy cold, blueness of limbs/body; desires to be fanned.

< warmth, depletion	> eructations
< dissipation; pressure of clothes	**> cool air**
< extreme temps, cold air, humid	> elevating feet

Caulophyllum

False pains, very rigid os; **severe spasmodic pains without progress**; pains flag from long continuance and exhaustion; thirst and fever; **erratic pains**, drawing, weak, irregular pains; pains in bladder and legs; uterine atony; **commonly indicated in pregnancy**.

< pregnancy, open air, PM
< suppressed menses

< cold	> warmth
< noise (labor pains)	

Chamomilla

Spasmodic, distressing pains, patient cannot bear them, wants to get away from them; fretful, **peevish and cross**; cannot return a civil answer; is spiteful; cries out sharply; tearing pains in back and down inner side of legs; **refuses what is offered**; hot and thirsty with pain; oversensitive, **moves about due to the pain** (Puls).

< anger, night	> being carried
< cold, damp air	> heat, sweating

< coffee, alcohol	> cold applications
< being spoken to	

China

Much blood loss; fainting; fits or convulsions; pain ceases with loss of vital fluids; patient cannot bear to be touched during the pains; weak, oversensitive; nervous; desires to be fanned (Carbo v), fresh air; cold skin and sweat; ringing in ears.

< vital fluid loss	> hard pressure
< touch, noise, jarring	> loose clothing
< cold, wind, drafts	
< eating fruit, milk	

Cimicifuga

After pains of childbirth, patient is **very sensitive to pain**; intolerant of the pains; **pains which run from hip to hip**; intense, heavy backache, pain shoots up and down anterior surface of thighs; **soreness of muscles**, especially after labor; pains > with bending double (Coloc, Nux v); false labor pains; patient faints from the pain (Nux v, Puls); **weak labor pains**, which extend to the groin; **spasm of the os during labor**; may have depression with a sense of impending evil; mania may follow cessation of pains; **subinvolution of the uterus**, prolapse.

Cocculus

Spasmodic **irregular paralytic pain**, in small of back, hard pain, then after a long interval some lighter ones; much headache; **numb, paralyzed feeling in** lower limbs; **trembling**, **spinal weakness**; clutching in uterus; nausea.

< motion; pain; noise
< loss of sleep; exertion
< touch; anxiety; cold
< open air

Conium

Tumors of breast or uterus; pains spasmodic; vertigo on turning in bed; spasms of os; **stony hardness**.

< seeing moving objects	> letting part hang down
< exertion, injury, PM	
< cold, sexual excesses	

Cuprum met

Violent spasmodic pains at irregular intervals with **severe cramps in lower extremities**, or in fingers and toes only; great restlessness between pains; cramps and spasms; hypersensitive; uneasy; nervous; sensation of loss of consciousness; tense abdomen; clonic spasms during pregnancy, patient becomes insensible to light and labor pains cease; after pains in women who have borne many children.

< anger, motion, vomiting	> cold drinks
< loss of sleep; touch	> pressure over heat
< suppressions	
< hot weather	

Gelsemium

Cutting pains in abdomen from front and below, upward and backward, rendering every labor pain useless; thick, **rigid os**, dread of falling; confused; **thirstless**; heavy, sore uterus; **drowsiness**; **apathetic**; pains insufficient, ceasing (similar to Caulophyllum), exhausted, anticipation brings on symptoms; tremulous excitement, **drooping eyelids**, **weakness of extraocular motion**.

< emotions, shock, surprise	> profuse urination
< spring, humid, fog, muggy	> sweating
< gas, tobacco	> shaking, alcohol
	> mental effort

Hyoscyamus

Delirium; startings and jerkings all over face; **spasmodic pains**, contracted os; mania; convulsions.

< fright; jealousy	> sitting up
< touch, injury, cold	
< sleep	

Ignatia

Deep sighs and sadness; takes a deep breath to breathe at all; hysterical symptoms; weak or ceasing labor pains (consider possible rigid os); moody, changeful; pain shoots up rectum; absorbed in grief; **oversensitive**, **nervous**, **alert**.

< grief, worry, chagrin	> change of position
< fright, shock; consolation	> lying on part
< open and cold air	> urination
< touch; odors; coffee	> alone; pressure

Ipecac

Constant nausea (Tab), sharp, cutting pain about the umbilicus to the uterus; **no thirst**, nausea not > with vomiting; **ineffectual vomiting**.

< warmth; damp	> open air
< overeating	
< heat and cold	

Kali carb

Pains begin in back to the buttocks; sharp cutting pains across lumbar region, arresting labor pains; **patient is disturbed by sharp stitching pains**; back and legs give out; wants her back pressed on; walks about and holds her low back; back labor pains.

< cold, air, exertion	> warmth, open air
< 2–3 AM	> sitting with elbows on knees
< lying on painful side	
< fluid loss, after labor	

Lycopodium

Keeps in motion with paroxysms of pain; spasmodic contraction of the os; repeating or alternating symptoms; frequent urge to urinate; pains go upward from right to left.

< pressure of clothes	> warm drinks
< warmth, waking	> cold applications
< 4–8 PM	> motion, eructations
< eating to satiety; oysters	> urinating

Magnesia mur

Labor pains interrupted by hysterical spasms; liver remedy; for women who have a history of indigestion and uterine diseases.

< lying on right side	> hard pressure, hanging down
< night; noise; milk	> bent; gentle motion
	> cool, open air

Natrum mur

Very **sad and foreboding**; feeble pains; ceasing slow progress; bearing-down pains (Sep); prolapsis of the uterus; Nat mur mentals.

< heat, 9–11 AM	> open air, cool bath
< sympathy, exertion of eyes	> sweating, rest
	> deep breathing

Nux moschata

Very drowsy, sleepy; **fainting spells**; slow and feeble pains; **dry mouth with no thirst**; delirium.

< cold, bath, damp, etc.	> moist heat, warm room
< pregnancy, excitement	> dry weather
< mental exertion; shock	
< airing	

Nux vomica

Every pain causes vesical and rectal tenesmus and fainting; **ineffectual urging**; debility from use of narcotics, alcohol, coffee; **urge to move bowels with each contraction**; sensation as if a ball in the rectum (Sepia); pains > bending double (Cimic).

Platina

Very painful sensitivity of vagina, external genitals; interrupts labor pains; spasmodic, painful, inefficient labor pains; her thoughts horrify her; disordered sense of proportion; irregular spasms; pains all on left side; haughty.

< touch; emotions	> walking in cool air; sun

Pulsatilla

Inertia uteri; pains excite palpitation, suffocating and fainting spells; wants doors and windows open; **no thirst**; very slow labor; helps with abnormal presentations; patient gets up and walks around; emotional, **weepy**, mild, **changing symptoms**, alternately happy and sad; gets stuck at various stages of labor; air hunger.

< warmth, wet feet	**> cold**, **open air**
< evening, rest, lying	> erect posture
< beginning motion	**> crying**; walking
< rich food, fat	

Ruta

Lame and sore all over; for any damage or over-stretching of ligaments (see indications under back pains); weak contractions; < after labor.

< overexertion; lying	> lying on back
< sitting; damp; wet	> warmth, motion
< eye strain	

Secale

Weak cachectic women; debilitated from bleeding or **from frequent and repeated child-bearing** (Sep); weak, suppressed or distressing pains; fainting, **do not give in material dose**, causes contraction of the os; cramps in hands, legs, feet; bearing down with coldness; inert uterus; hourglass contraction of uterus; **external icy cold but burning hot internal**, **< being covered**.

< warmth, covering	> cold; bathing; uncovering
< loss of fluid; rocking; forcible extension	

Sepia

Shuddering with pains; wants to be covered so she can bear pains easier; induration felt upon neck of uterus; shooting pains travel upward; spasmodic contraction of os; indifference to birth and family; nausea at thought or smell of food (Colch); involuntary weeping or laughter; uterine prolapse, **crosses legs to keep it in**; **extreme dragging-down feeling in pelvis**, especially after birth.

< cold, AM & PM
< before menses

> violent motions
> warmth, cold drinks

RIGID OS

Antimonium tart

Rigid os with much nausea and dyspnea; history of subacute chronic pelvic inflammatory disease.

Caulophyllum

False pains with a very rigid os; severe spasmodic contractions; pains become weaker as patient becomes more exhausted.

Gelsemium

False pains; cramps in various parts of abdomen, pains from front & below, upward & backward; **os is round**; **hard**, **thick**; **rigid**; will not dilate; face is flushed, dark; apathetic with droopy, dull mentation.

Ignatia

If Nux fails and Ignatia mentals present; deep sighing and breathing in order to catch her breath.

Lobelia

Thick, leathery, unyielding cervix; nausea with each pain, violent dyspnea.

Nux vomica

Pains in loins; constant urge to stool; vesicle and rectal pain with contractions; tetanic rigidity of os.

Passiflora

Tetanic rigidity of os; hysterical subjects.

Pulsatilla

Uterine inertia; spasmodic pains with suffocation and fainting; no thirst; slow labor and dilation of the os.

Veratrum viride

Rigid os with threatened convulsions; plethora; pulse full, hard and quick; congested head; chest.

SPASM OF OS

Aconite

Much heat and dryness of the of the vagina and os; os is contracted and will not dilate further; patient is restless, fearful and anxious.

Actea spicata

Severe spasm with ineffectual pains; os is at one time dilating and at another has suddenly closed; patient is nervous and melancholy.

Lachesis

Contracted os with throat and heart symptoms; women near menopause.

POST PARTUM—APGAR

Aconite

For fear, fright or shock of delivery; child will have a frightened or terrified look on its face; use if APGAR is in the 1-to-4 range.

Arnica

Birth trauma, bruised feeling or **observations of bruising**, following a difficult delivery through a narrow canal; soft tissue contusions due to a large baby or prolonged labor (for both mother and child); baby is in shock-like state, stunned; can give to mom if baby isn't delivered yet; good to use if skull is deformed when coming through the canal or later if moulding does not take place. Consider **Bellis per** for mother following birth.

Antimonium tart

Infant is **blue** and **pale** with cold, clammy skin; **nostrils may be dilated but not necessarily active**; asphyxia due to meconium, cord prolapse with drowsiness; **rattling** of respiration; APGAR of 1-to-4.

Arsenicum alb

APGAR in the 1-to-4 range, **difficult or decreased respirations** (Carbo veg); decreased heart rate, pale, flaccid child; **child struggles for air, appears anxious, fearful** (Aconite); consider if meconium aspiration, extreme prostration.

Laurocerasus

Blue babies due to asphyxia; cyanosis with difficulty breathing which may be < sitting up; face is blue and the **child is gasping for breath**, may be foaming at the mouth, twitching of the facial muscles; extremities are cold, clammy which is not > by warmth, and there may be clubbing of the fingers; mitral regurgitation; infant may appear fearful, anxious and is **> with head lying low**.

See section under **SHOCK/COLLAPSE** for additional remedies.

UTERINE DISPLACEMENTS
Prolapse, Anteversion, Retroversion

Aesculus

Pain about the sacro-iliac symphysis (dull pain); cannot walk due to back giving out; constipation and hemorrhoids.

< walking, urinating	> cool open air and bathing
< after stool; stooping	> bleeding; kneeling
< waking	> continued exertion

Aletris

Prolapse of uterus; **obstinate nausea and vomiting of pregnancy**; false pains; debility; tendency to abort; pain with stool; heaviness of pelvis.

< loss of fluids	> passing flatus
	> bending backward

Belladonna

Uterine displacements, pressure as though everything were **coming down through external genitals**; especially in AM; heat and dryness of vagina; sharp pains come and go suddenly in pelvis and back; back so sore patient can hardly move.

< heat of sun, 3 PM
< drafts on head, washing head
< check sweat; light; noise
< jarring; pressure; touch

> light covering
> bending backward
> bed rest

Calcarea carb

Uterine displacements; feet and legs feel as if patient had on wet socks; **vertigo on going up stairs**; shortness of breath and must sit and rest; **constant wearing ache in vagina and rectum**, melancholy in PM.

< cold, wet, change of weather
< exertion , mental, physical
< pressure of clothes
< milk
< anxiety

Calcarea phos

Especially for retroversion; **every cold causes rheumatic pains** in joints and elsewhere.

< touch
< cold, wet
< heat of room

> bathing, eating
> open air
> local heat, uncovering

Caulophyllum

Prolapse and retroversion; uterine congestion with fullness; heaviness and tension in hypogastrium; drawing pains in groin; **threatened miscarriage**; false labor pains.

< pregnancy
< suppressed menses
< open air; in PM

Cimicifuga

Prolapse and retroversion: sensation of weight and bearing-down in uterine region with heaviness and torpor in lower extremities; **neuralgia or rheumatoid diathesis**; history of dysmenorrhea and abortion.

Conium

Induration and prolapsus; **vertigo when turning over in bed**; **intermittent urination**, sore breasts, enlarged and painful; history of ovarian problems; cancer.

< seeing moving objects	> letting part hang down
< alcohol, sexual excesses	
< after exertion, injury	
< night; cold	
< old age; lying	

Helonias

Deep, undefined depression and sensation of prolapse, soreness and weight in uterus; **consciousness of a womb**; bleeding and threatened abortion after lifting the least weight or moving about; albuminuria, pruritus pudendi; similar to Conium.

< fatigue; labor; abortion; stooping	> if busy, diversions
< pregnancy	> holding abdomen
< pressure of clothes	

Kali carb

Heavy aching pain in small of back; stitching pains in uterus; dry bronchial cough; wakes at 3 AM feeling bad all over.

< cold air, water, drafts	> warmth, open air
< loss of fluids	> sitting with elbows on knees
< winter; exertion	
< 2–3 AM, lying on painful or left side	

Lilium tig

All displacements; **bearing-down as if everything would come through the vagina**, **places hands on vulva to prevent it**; severe neuralgic pain in uterus; all her troubles began with a miscarriage; pains and bearing-down seem to extend and drag from shoulders and chest downward.

< warmth of room	> cool, fresh air
< motion, miscarriages	> when busy
< walking, standing	> lying on left side
< consolation	> pressure, crossing legs

Lycopodium

Especially retroversion; flatulent dyspepsia and constipation; **terrific pain in back previous to urination, with relief as the very hot urine flows**; red sand in urine; cutting pain across hypogastrium from right to left; repeating or alternating symptoms.

< pressure of clothes	> warm drinks, food
< warmth, wind	> cold applications
< awakening	> motion; eructations
< indigestion; **4–8 PM**	> urinating

Mercurius

All displacements; cold clammy sweat on thighs every evening; deep, sore pain in pelvis; abdomen feels weak as if it must be helped up; itching of genitals; wide variety of symptoms; sensitive to drafts on head.

< night, sweating	> moderate temperatures
< lying on right side	
< heated, bed or fire	
< cloudy, damp weather, heat and cold	

Murex

Especially retroversion; sore pain in womb as if cut by a sharp instrument; nervous temperament; strong will and cheerful disposition; pain on right side from abdomen to chest; nymphomania; must cross limbs (Sep).

< touch, in sun	> before menses
< sitting, abortion	> eating

Natrum mur

Prolapsus; pushing towards genitals every AM; has to sit to avoid prolapse; **awakens in AM with violent headache:** itching of external parts and falling off of hair; constipation with fissures; imagines robbers in house.

< with sun, 9–11 AM	> open air, sweating
< after menses, alternate days	> cool bathing, rest
< heat	> before breakfast
< exertion, eyes, mental	> deep breathing
< violent emotions	
< sympathy	

Nux vomica

Uterine deviations from lifting or straining; agg. from walking or standing, dyspepsia, constipations, piles; **urinates frequently but a little at a time**, headache and backache; wakes 3 AM and cannot get to sleep.

< early AM	> free discharges
< cold, open air, uncovering, drafts	> naps, rest
< high living, coffee, alcohol	> wrapping head
< overeating, purgatives	> hot drinks; moisture
< mental exertion	
< slight noises, odors, touch	
< pressure of clothes	

Phosphorus

Tall, slender redheads; plethoric women who pass long, narrow, hard, dry stools; stitching pain upward from vagina cut through the pelvis; heat running up the back; emptiness and weakness in abdomen.

< lying on left side; painful side or back	> eating, sleep, cold
< emotions; evening	> rubbing
< cold—hands, open air	> sitting up
< warm ingesta	

< sexual excesses
< weather—sudden changes, windy, cold, thunderstorms

Platina

Great sensitiveness of genitals and continual pressure and bearing-down; body is cold and numb; constipation—stool soft and sticks to the anus like clay; melancholy or peculiar proud, defiant mood, feels more important or above others; hard, black, difficult stools.

< emotions—sexual, coition	> walking in cool air
< touch	> sunshine

Podophyllum

Prolapsus of uterus and anus, especially after confinement; sensation as if genitals would come out during stool; constipation, liver troubles; AM diarrhea; burning pain in small of back.

< early AM, eating	> stroking liver
< hot weather, motion	> lying on abdomen
< dentition	

Pulsatilla

Cries easily, is dependent; very bad taste in mouth in AM; pressure in abdomen and small of back like a stone; disposition of lower limbs to go to sleep when sitting; ineffectual desire for stool (Nux v), **thirstless with dry mouth**; symptoms change, drift.

< warm room, bed, clothes	> cold, fresh air
< getting feet wet, rest, PM	> uncovering, erect posture
< beginning motion	> gentle motion
< rich foods; fats	> after crying
< before menses; lying on left side	

Ruta

Prolapse of rectum with every stool, especially after confinement; tendency to constipation, but may be alternating with mucus; sensation of constriction higher up in the rectum; **protrusion of rectum** with stooping, after childbirth.

Sepia

Especially retroversion; pressing in uterus; oppressive breathing; sensation as if everything will come out of vagina, **crosses legs to prevent it**; constipation, with **sensation of weight in the anus, not > with evacuation**; swollen labia.

< cold air	> violent motion
< sexual excesses, before menses	> warmth
< pregnancy, abortion	> cold drinks
< AM & PM	

RETAINED PLACENTA

Belladonna

Red face and eyes; great distress and moaning; **much heat and dryness of vagina** (Acon), profuse flow of hot blood that coagulates rapidly; slightest jar causes suffering and restlessness.

< heat, drafts on head	> light covering
< light; noise; jarring	> bending backward
< touch; motion	> resting bed

Cantharis

Burning pains in pelvis and back; fever, vomiting; great anguish with discharge of fluid blood and clots in equal parts with every pain; swelling of lips of os; may have an **intense desire to urinate**.

< urinating; bright objects	> warmth, rest
< drinking, sound of water	
< touch	

Cimicifuga

For women with rheumatic affections, distressing, tearing pain, uterine atony; gloomy feeling, low spirits; oversensitive.

< menses, labor	> warm wraps, open air
< damp air, wind	> pressure, eating
< cold drafts, hot and cold	> continued motion
< sitting	

Gelsemium

Cutting pains in lower abdomen running upward and/or backward; aching, tired, heavy, weak, sore, confused, droopy.

< emotions, dread, shock	> profuse urination
< heat of summer	> sweating
< spring, humid, foggy weather	> shaking; alcohol
	> mental effort

Pulsatilla

Most often used; uterine inertia; **spasmodic retention**, intermittent flow of blood; restless; desires fresh air; weepy; mild, yielding disposition; **thirstless**.

< warm rooms, evenings	> cold, fresh, open air
< rest, beginning to move	> erect posture
< rich foods, fat	> gentle motion; crying

Sabina

Intense after-pains, with discharge of fluid blood and clots in equal parts with pain; pain or uneasiness in sacrum and pubes with some sensation of motion in abdomen, pain from lumbar to pubes, or in reverse.

< night; heat	> cold, cool, open air
< foggy weather	
< exercise, moving around	

Secale

Constant sensation of bearing; passive hemorrhage; parts seem relaxed with absence of uterine action; in thin women; wants abdomen uncovered; numbness, tingling, twitching; icy cold external, burning hot internal.

< warmth, loss of fluid	> cold, uncovering
< covers	> rocking, forcible extension

Sepia

Little, sharp, shooting pain in cervix, sometimes with burning; indifference; dragging, bearing-down feeling; hot hands, cold feet.

< cold air, wind	> violent motion
< before menses, AM & PM	> warmth, cold drinks

POSTPARTUM HEMORRHAGE

Aconite

Active arterial bleeding; **fear of death**, **restless** but is unable to sit up in bed.

Apocynum

Uterine bleeding with great irritability of the stomach; flux with large clots and shreds; **urinary and dropsical complications**, fainting; thirst, vomits every drink; cannot sweat.

< cold weather, drinks	> warmth
< uncovering, lying	

Argentum nit

Confusion, head pain, agg. by least motion; short time seems forever; everything done seems to take forever; belching relieves distress; craves sugar, craves fresh air; violent pains like splinters, uterine hemorrhages, up to two weeks after menses.

< anxiety, suspense	> cool air; bath
< in shut room	> hard pressure
< sugar, drinking	> motion

Arnica

After a full shock, concussion or fatigue; constant bright red or clotted flux with or without pain; nausea in pit of stomach; hot head with cool extremities; feels sore and bruised in uterine region (Bellis); hemorrhagic tendency; fears being struck, instant death; must uncover but it chills her.

< bruises, shock, jarring
< overexertion; labor
< touch; motion

> lying with head low
> lying outstretched

Arsenicum alb

Lancinating, burning pains; very restless; sudden great weakness; thin secretions; cadaveric odor; agonizing fear of death; insatiable burning thirst for cold water; heat as if hot water in veins or waves of icy cold in veins.

< cold drinks, food
< exertion
< after midnight, 3 AM
< eruptions
< lying on part

> hot food, drinks and applications
> motion, elevating head
> company, sweating

Belladonna

Profuse discharge of **bright, red-hot blood with downward pressure**, as if all would escape; pain in back as if it would break; blood coagulates easily, is sometimes offensive; **flowing between and after pains**; hot face and head, congested red head and eyes; restless; talks fast; head sensitive to cold and drafts.

< light, noise, motion
< touch, company, pressure

> light covering
> bending backward
> bed rest

Bryonia

Dark red bleeding with pain in the back, splitting headache; dry mouth and lips, thirst; nausea and vertigo on sitting up or raising head; **averse to motion.**

< motion, any
< dry heat or cold
< becoming hot; hot room
< eating; touch

> lying on painful part
> cool open air; quiet
> drawing knees up
> heat to inflamed parts

Calcarea carb

Plethoric women with light hair, usually menstruate too often, too much and too long; vertigo on stooping, going up stairs; cold, damp feet; sour discharges.

< cold air, bathing
< exertion, physical, mental
< pressure of clothes
< milk

Cantharis

Bleeding of uterus with great irritation of bladder neck; cutting, burning pains during frequent efforts to urinate, can urinate a few drops only; **burning thirst but averse to liquids**; bloody urine.

< urinating
< cold drinks
< sound of water
< touch

> warmth, rest

Carbo veg

Passive hemorrhage; cold and deathly pale, excessive prostration; burning pains across sacrum; excessive flatus; itching of vulva and anus; dark oozing bleeding; dusky face, icy cold; **> cool air blown into face**.

< warmth, depletions
< air, open air
< pressure of clothes
< cold weather, wind
< cooling off

> eructations, **cool air**
> elevating feet

Caulophyllum

Profuse bleeding from relaxed or feebly contracting uterus—after a hasty labor; passive oozing hemorrhage; fretful, nervous, excitable.

< pregnancy
< suppressed menses
< open air; evening

Chamomilla

Irascibility or spiteful irritability; flow is dark, coagulated, black, fetid, lumpy with frequent discharge of colorless urine; tearing pains in legs; violent labor pains; blood flows by fits and starts at irregular intervals; oversensitive.

< anger; night	> being carried; held
< cold air, wind	> mild weather
< coffee	> heat, sweating
	> cold applications

China

Bleeding due to uterine atony; **dark clots**, uterine spasm; **bleeds dark blood which is thin and watery**; loss of vital fluids causes fainting and syncope; **skin cold and blue**; twitching of muscles, heavy head, tinnitus, loss of sight, fainting, weak pulse; weak, oversensitive, very sensitive to drafts; nervous; **chilly** and wants lots of covers (opp Puls & Secale).

< loss of fluids, touch	> hard pressure
< noise; jars	> loose clothes
< open air, cold	
< fruit, milk	
< mental exertion	

Cimicifuga

Consider for bleeding if accompanied by **cramping pains**, **pains which run from hip to hip**; great intolerance to pains; the greater the flow of blood, the greater the pain; **nervous**, **excitable**, **fidgety**.

< labor; emotions	**> pressure**

Crocus

Dark, **stringy bleeding**, in dark or black strings, after walking, with or without pain; sensation of rolling or bounding in abdomen; often seen with post partum bleeding; rapidly changing symptoms; sensation as if something is alive, moving in various parts of the body; sudden mood changes from dark to gay.

< motion, heat

< pregnancy; looking at a fixed object

> open air

Erigeron

Profuse, bright-red bleeding, alarmingly increased at every movement (Sabina), with irritation of bladder and rectum; gushing bleeding; smarting; burning.

< rainy weather

Ferrum met

Bleeding, with fiery red face and hard full pulse; flow partly fluid and partly black clotted with violent labor-like pains; headache, vertigo, constipation, hot urine, great weakness; anemia; dilated veins.

< night; exertion

< loss of fluids; sweats

< heat and cold; sudden motion

> gentle motion

> leaning head on something

Ficus

Hemorrhages of any kind; bright red blood; desires to pass urine with much blood, sputum with blood; bearing-down pains in lower abdomen with uterine bleeding; weakness and restlessness; **use in 1x, low potency or in tincture form**.

Hamamelis

Passive hemorrhage with anemia; steady, slow, dark; painless flow; painful varicosities; sore veins; irritable; chilly; hemorrhoids.

< injury; pressure

< open air; cold or humid air

< jar, motion; touch

Hyoscyamus

Bleeding with spasms of whole body, with jerks or twitching of single limb; bright red continuous flow; delirium or mania; wants to escape, nervous wakefulness.

< full moon, storms, suppressions

Iodum

Hemorrhage with every stool, cutting in abdomen and pains in loins, small of back.

< heat; warm room	> cold, air, bathing
< exertion, night, rest	> motion, eating

Ipecac

Constant, **profuse**, **bright red flow**, or **flows in gushes**; bleeding clots quickly; with incessant nausea and vomiting; cutting pain about umbilicus; cold and pale, faint, gasps for breath; **good for after expulsion of child**, **placenta**, no thirst; nausea not > with vomiting.

< warmth; movement	> open air
< overeating	
< heat and cold	

Kali carb

Bleeding with stitching pain; pulse is small, soft, variable, intermittent; aversion to solitude.

< cold air, water, drafts	> warmth
< 2–3 AM	> sitting with elbows on knees
< lying on painful side, left side	> open air
< loss of fluids; after labor	

Lachesis

Paroxysms of pain in right ovary, relieved by a gush of blood; thin hemorrhages; dark particles; ascending sensations; left-sided to right side; loquacity; flushes of heat; rapid onset.

< after sleep, AM	> open air
< empty swallowing	> discharges
< slight touch; clothing	> cold drinks
	> hard pressure

Lycopodium

Profuse, protracted flowing; partly black, clotted partly bright red or serum: with labor-like pains until she faints; full of gas; repeating or alternating symptoms.

< clothing	> warm drinks, food
< warmth, awaking	> cold applications
< 4–8 PM, indigestion	> motion, eructations
	> urinating

Millefolium

Profuse, sudden, bright red fluid; bleeding after much exertion, esp, in plethoric women; use with China; painless bleeding.

< injury, violent motion	> bleeding, discharges

Nitric acid

Bleeding with violent pressure, as if everything were coming out vulva; with pain in small of back through hips and down thighs; hemorrhages easily, bright, bloody water; quarrelsome, delirious, angry, confusion; urine smells strong; acrid discharges; cracking of skin.

< slight touch, jar, motion, noise	> gliding motions; riding
< cold air, damp	> mild weather
< night; heat of bed	> steady pressure
< mental exertion	

Nux moschata

Dark, thick, **long-continued bleeding** (Ustilago), especially after abortion, with dry mouth and tongue; fainting, sleeplessness, hysteria; dry mouth with no thirst; drowsiness.

< cold, pregnancy	> moist heat, warm room
< emotions, excitement	> dry weather
< menses	
< jar, bruises	

Phosphorus

Bleeding after difficult labor, in tall, slim women with black or red hair; constipation; vicarious hemorrhage; human barometers (Merc); bright-red flowing blood; **craves cold drinks** vomits when warm.

< lying on left side or painful side	> eating; sleeping
< emotional causes, bathing, odors	> cold food, water
< cold hands, open air	> rubbing
< changes in weather	> sitting up
< AM & PM	

Platina

Profuse, **dark**, thick blood with pain in back extending to groin and excessive **sensibility of the genitals**, **black clots** or a thick tarry mass; sensation (with flow) as if the body were growing larger; contemptuous, arrogant.

< emotions, sexual, chagrin	> walking in cool air
< touch	

Pulsatilla

Intermittent black hemorrhage with clots; **alternates with labor pains**, mild, gentle weeping; wants doors and windows open; **thirstless**; changing symptoms; air hunger, **desires fresh air**.

< warm room, air, bed	> cold, fresh air
< evening; rest, beginning motion	> erect posture
< lying on left side	> gentle motion
< eating rich, fatty foods	> crying

Sabina

Dark, red hemorrhage **with dark clots in thin watery blood** (China); painless bleeding; forcing-down pain from sacrum to pubes; **least movement increases flow but walking decreases it**; **gushing** hot **watery blood**; patient can bleed for a long period of time (days to weeks) after birth; pain from pubes to sacrum; pain > passing clots; patient is anxious; seen in plethoric constitutions.

< night
< heat; bed; room; exercise

> cold, cool, open air
> passing clots of blood

Secale

Passive bleeding of dark, fetid, thin blood in feeble, cachectic women, have had many children; strong very painful bearing-down pains; desires air; does not want to be covered even though body is cold; uterine atony; cold external yet hot internal; **thirsty**. Several authors have touted the use of this medicine in tincture form, 10 drops in water for bleeding.

< warmth; covers

> cold bathing; uncovering
> rocking
> forcible extension

Sepia

Congestion with sensation of weight; pain in right groin; fine darting pain neck of uterus from below to up; feels better with drawing up limbs; icy cold paroxysms and flushes of heat; cold feet; painful all-gone feeling in pit of stomach; constipated; angry; sensitive; irritable.

< cold; air; wind
< pregnancy
< AM & PM

> violent motion
> warmth; cold drinks

Stramonium

Delirium with bleeding, excessive loquacity, singing, praying; strange ideas, hallucinations; drawing pains in limbs; dreads darkness.

< glistening objects; fright
< after sleep

> light; company
> warmth

Sulphur

Chronic bleeding, seems almost well then is worse; weakness, fainting, hunger, flushes of heat, hot head and cold feet; sore abdomen; craves fresh air.

< bathing; suppressions

> open air; motion

< heated; bed
< exertion
< 11 AM; full moon

> warm applications
> sweating; dry heat

Trillium

Active hemorrhage; **thick, dark, clotted blood after confinement or abortion**, great prostration; frequently used; gushing blood; pubic pain extends to sacrum.

< motion

> exertion in open air
> tight bandage around hips
> bending forward

Ustilago

Chronic passive bleeds; slow persistent **oozing** of **dark blood** with small black clots; dark semifluid but not watery blood; uterine inertia; bleeds slowly; **spongy cervix**; dry, hot skin; metrorrhagia from labor, bright red, offensive, putrid; constant flow during and after labor; inertia of uterus and softening of os during labor.

< touch; motion

MASTITIS

Belladonna

Breasts feel heavy, **hot** and sore and **show red streaks radiating from the areola**; pulsating pains which come on quickly; generally not as painful; patient is thirstless, lethargic; more right-sided.

Bryonia

Hardness of the breasts which feel **hot** (Bell) **and painful** but are not as red as Belladonna; ill feeling, especially if she gets up or moves; **thirst for cold drinks** and may be accompanied by a stitching headache; consider using before Aconite.

< movement
< heat

> cold, cold applications

Hepar sulph

The remedy to consider if **suppuration is inevitable**; various authors suggest not giving it too soon as it may accelerate the process, but to give it in low dose often once the suppuration has begun.

Phosphorus

Inflammation of the breasts with red spots, streaks and stitching (Bry), cutting pains; **knotty abscesses or fistulous ulcerations** which burn, sting and have an offensive watery discharge; more left-sided.

Phytolacca

Painful swelling of the breast with chills followed by fever; hardness of the breast (Bry) with many painful nodes; abscesses with many fistulous openings, watery, fetid, ichorous pus which may dry and cake solid; tremendous pain which radiates from the breast in every direction; is useful in most every stage of mastitis and can be used both internally and externally in hot packs.

Silicea

Abscess which is slow to form; fistulous ulceration which discharges a thin, watery, offensive pus; many areas of discharge which may open into one drainage tract; slow to heal; **patient is chilly**, **weak** and craves the heat.

LACTATION

Acetic acid

Large and profuse **flow of milk** which is normal in quality.

Borax

Stitching and aching pains in the breast with a **scanty flow of milk**, better with compression; galactorrhea; pains in opposite breast with nursing; empty feeling in breasts after nursing.

Lac caninum

Drying-up of milk, galactorrhea or scanty production of milk post partum; **breasts are swollen and painful and < with jarring**,

touch, condition is > with menses; good remedy for mastitis; **erratic pains which change from side to side**, consider **Lac defloratum** to restore a scanty flow of milk.

Pulsatilla

Flow of milk is slow, **scanty**, suppressed; secretion of milk during menses; **weeps with nursing**; swelling of the breasts after child is no longer nursing; **milk is thin and watery**; breasts may be swollen and painful which makes nursing difficult; may be associated with rheumatic pains; patient is **tearful** and **thirstless**.

FAILURE TO NURSE

Aethusa

Vomiting of milk as soon as it is swallowed or about an hour later, in large curds or as frothy matter, may be followed by weakness and a deep sleep; **intolerance of milk** with nausea and vomiting; vomiting or projectile vomiting with sweating and weakness; weakness of children who can hardly hold up their heads; diarrhea of yellow, green and slimy material (Mag carb).

Symptoms in Kent's Repertory	**Page**
Genital-F, Abortion/tendency to	714
Genital-F, Contractions, os, spasmodic	716
Genital-F, Contractions, hourglass	716
Genital-F, Itching, pregnancy, during	720
Genital-F, leukorrhea, pregnancy	722
Genital-F, Pain, bearing down uterus	735
Genital-F, Pain, griping, labor-like	739
Genital-F, Pain, extending to back & hips	739
Genital-F, Pain, false	739
Genital-F, Pain, ineffectual/irregular	739
Genital-F, Pain, spasmodic	740
Genital-F, Prolapsus, uterus	743
Genital-F, Placenta, retained	743

OTITIS MEDIA/EARACHES

Earaches are commonly seen in children from as early as 6 months of age until 7 years. Adults are also affected but less commonly. Earaches can be broken down into three types of otitis: serous, infective and external. Both infective and serous otitis often follow **upper respiratory infections**, but are also seen in children who are bottle-fed while lying down and those who have been exposed to cold, windy weather. A strong association with chronic earaches and food allergies has been made, especially milk, other dairy products and wheat.

An acute **infective earache** will more likely occur during the winter months and may be announced with a high fever, throbbing of the ear, irritability, tugging at the ear and pain. Fever may also not be present and the person affected may be lethargic and complain of not feeling well. If a discharge is seen from the ear canal, then the eardrum has ruptured and there will be some hearing loss for a period of time until it has been able to repair itself.

Serous otitis is accompanied by a sense of fullness, hearing loss, ringing in the ears and little or no pain. In this condition, there is a buildup of fluid behind the ear drum which causes the hearing loss. If left untreated, it can develop into an infective condition.

External otitis is characterized by an inflammation of the external ear canal. Otherwise known as swimmer's ear, it is caused by repeated wetting of the canal which allows for bacterial or fungal growth.

Aconite

First stage; intense attack after exposure to **dry**, **cold winds**; **bright red ears**, **high fever** (104°F), dry skin; rapid pulse; **sharp pain**; **very sensitive to noise**; one cheek red, one pale; much fear, thinks he will die; **anxious**, **restless**; increased thirst for cold drinks; child holds ear, screams with pain; no effusion or liquid, tympanic membrane intact (not bulging); sensation as if a drop of water in left ear; **burning thirst**.

< violent emotions; **fright**; **shock**	> open air; repose
< sleeping in sun	> warm sweat
< cold wind; dry wind	
< pressure; touch	
< noise; light; during dentition	
< night, in bed, lying on side	
< warm room; mucus	
< tobacco smoke	

Belladonna (2)

Local congestion, ear and head; exposed parts dry but perspires on covered parts, legs, etc.; **dilated pupils** (Agnus); **throbbing** carotids, eardrums, entire body; pulse is hard; cerebral symptoms if severe; tympanic membrane is red, bulging, prominent blood vessels; hot head and cold body; **sudden onset** of pain in ear and just as suddenly it leaves; tearing pain in middle and external ear; swollen parotid gland; **pain causes delirium**; **child cries out in sleep**; pain synchronous with heart beat; autophony—hearing one's voice in ear; hematoma auris; sensitive to loud noises, hearing very acute; **throbbing**, **sharp**, **shooting**, **cutting** pains; rolls head, **jerks during sleep**; pains go downward from head, thirst; wasted, does not want to move; **little thirst anxiety or fear**; **no thirst with fever**.

< heat of sun, if heated	> light covering
< afternoon (3 PM); night	> bending backward
< drafts, on head, hair cut, washing head	> bed rest
< after taking cold; cold air	> semi-erect
< light; **checked sweating**; **noise**	
< jarring; touch; company	
< motion; pressure; hanging down	

Calcarea carb (3)

Throbbing, cracking in ears; stitching & pulsating pain as if something would pass out; scrofulous inflammation with **mucopurulent otorrhea**, **enlarged glands**; difficulty and perversions of hearing; sensitive to cold about ears and neck; takes cold easily; **pro-fuse, often sour discharges**; internal heat with external sweat, coldness; sad, apathetic, indolent, **apprehensive**; craves eggs, Calcarea constitutions; milk disagrees.

< cold; **air**, **bathing**, wet	> dry climates, weather
< change of weather; standing	> lying on painful side
< exertion, mental, physical	> sneezing
< ascending	
< dentition; puberty	
< pressure of clothes	
< milk; awaking, anxiety	

Chamomilla (3)

Affects nerves; ears red, hot, violent pain which causes screaming; thirsty, restless, **irritable**, fretful; does not know what they want; nothing appeases; **much pain then very irritable**; **one cheek red**, **one pale**; ringing in ears; stitching pain, ears feel stopped; ***mental calmness contraindicates Cham;*** night sweats; **wants to be held**, **carried**; sensitive to cold wind on ear (Hepar); hot and thirsty with pains; **earaches from teething** (Calc-p, Terebinth).

< anger, **night**, **dentition**	**> being carried**
< cold, air, damp	> mild weather; heat
< wind; taking cold	> sweating; cold applications
< coffee; narcotics; alcohol	
< open air	

Ferrum phos (2)

First stage before exudate; **wet cold**; **pulsating**, throbbing pain; whole face flushed; tympanic membrane is slightly hyperemic, hiatus slightly red; **high fever**, ***few symptoms;*** sticking, throbbing pain; humming in ear—local hypertension; tender mastoid; blood vessels enlarged over membrane, red bulging; no thirst; tinnitus < lying; face pales and reddens alternately; fevers; use when Belladonna fails; thirsty; little anxious restlessness.

< night (4–6 AM); motion	> cold; lying down
< noise; cold air	

< checked sweat
< touch; right side

Hepar sulph (3)

Starts left to right; mucus, pus in ear; must get it out; thick, white, creamy discharge after suppuration; thin, offensive, smelly, green discharge **that gets <** after discharging; deafness due to scarlet fever; sharp, **stitching pain**; may have sore throat with pain to ear while swallowing; tenderness over mastoid; whizzing, throbbing in ear with decreased hearing; mastoiditis; **chilly**, **oversensitive**, bad tempers, irritability; **sweats easily**, with no relief; **covers ear and/or head**; thirsty.

< cold, dry, **air**, **winter,drafts wind**	**> heat;wraps**
	> head wrapped
< least, **uncovering**; **touch**	> moist heat
< exertion; lying on painful part	**> damp weather**
< night; noise	> after eating

Lycopodium (3)

Thick, yellow, offensive discharge; otorrhea, deafness with or without ringing in the ears; after scarlatina; **humming and roaring with deafness**; every noise causes peculiar echo in ear; repeating or alternating symptoms; **awakes angry**; **sensitive** and fearsome; **aversion to being alone**; pains cause anger, jerking; sudden onset of symptoms; **much noisy flatulence**; symptoms go right to left; **craves everything warm**, chilly.

< pressure of clothes	**> warm drinks**, food, etc.
< warmth; awaking; wind	> cold applications
< eating, to satiety, oysters	> motion; eructations
< indigestion; **4–8 PM**	> urinating
< above to downward	> after midnight
< warm applications except at throat	

Mercurius (3)

Follows Hepar well; otitis with swollen parotid, **offensive breath**, mucus, perspiration; **moist tongue and mouth with thirst**; bleeding of canal after physical exam; deafness > blowing nose, swallowing;

deafness after measles or swollen tonsils; thin, acrid discharge or **thick yellow-green**; stinging pain, sticking; **bleeding**; sensation as if cold water coming out of ear; ears itch; chronic otitis; **fetid**, **bloody discharge**; boils in external ear; pain sticks at one point; **metallic** or salty taste; pains into ears from teeth; **easy**, **profuse sweating**; deafness with becoming heated; aggravated by extremes of temperature; weakness, exhaustion, tremulous, **thirsty**, chilly.

< **night**, air
< **lying on right side**
< **heated**; **sweating**
< **drafts**, to head
Sensitive to: cold damp weather, changes in temperature
< warm room, bed

> moderate temperatures
> after sweating, wet feet

Pulsatilla (3)

Can be 2rd, 3rd or chronic stage; if unsure what to give, give Puls; suppressed cold; gets feet wet; deafness after whooping cough, measles, scarlet fever; external ear red, tragus has sores—1st stages; feels as if something trying to get out; **copious**, **thick**, **bland**, **yellow-green discharge**; stuffed-pus sensation (2nd stage); hears roaring and is synchronous with pulse, chilly but not cold; fretful, whiny; tearful; increased pain the more cold they become; feel less chilled by going outside; discharge is offensive; **changing symptoms**; nightly earaches; **thirstless.**

< **warmth**, **air**, **room**, bed
< getting feet wet
< **suppressions**; **evening**; **rest**
< **beginning motion**, **lying on side**
< **rich foods**; **fats**, ice, eggs
< **puberty**, after eating
< allowing feet to hang down

> **cold**; **fresh open air**
> uncovering; gentle motion
> **erect posture**
> weeping; being held

Silicea (3)

Similar to Merc but later, do not give after Merc; slow discharge (2 weeks); necrosis of ear bones, mastoid; thin, acrid, fetid discharge, slightly curdy; perforations that refuse to heal; pain goes from inward to out; itching; tingling in Eustachian tube; bores finger in ear; loses hearing quickly and comes back with loud sounds; does not mind having ear examined; much perspiration; sensitive; **roaring in ears**; **very sensitive to noise**, pain or cold; **foul foot sweats**, **chilly**; **sweat**, profuse, head, at night; fair complexion; mental acuteness with physical weakness; **thirsty**; **ill effects of vaccination**.

< cold; **air**; **drafts**; damp	**> warm**, **wraps to head**
< uncovering; checked sweat	> profuse urination
< change of moon; night; alcohol	> wrapping ear
< mental exertion	> wet or humid weather
Sensitive to excitement, light, noise, jarring spine	
< bathing; open air; motion	
< in AM; lying down	

Sulphur (3)

Ill effects from suppression of an otorrhea; sensitive to odors; deafness preceded by exceedingly sensitive hearing; deafness due to catarrh; whizzing in ears; **deficient reaction**; **red orifices**; **local throbbing**, **burning or congestion**; foul, acrid or blood-streaked discharge; hot head, cold feet; **thirsty**, chilly.

< suppressions; **bathing**	> open air; motion
< heated; **exertion**; **in bed**	> warm applications
< speaking; atmosphere changes	> sweat; dry heat
< rest; night	> lying on right side

Consider:

Bacillinum

Purulent bilateral otitis with discharge that is continuous, temperature 101–103; > hot; discharge is yellow and sticky; child light-complexioned, blond, chubby; tends to be constipated, decreased appetite; perspires on head (Calc.).

Baryta carb

Hard of hearing; **crackling noise**; **swollen painful glands around ears**; reverberation on blowing nose; **slow**, **inept**, **and backwards** children; thirsty; **chilly**.

Capsicum (2)

Otitis with ruptured membrane; very deep infection, swollen mastoid, red, shiny, tender, chronic discharge; **mastoid abscess**; external ear very red; **tenderness**, **soreness of mastoid**, **swelling and pain of mastoid**; **homesick**; feels sorry for himself; < night, cold air; > heat, continued motion (slow).

Carbo veg (2)

Otorrhea following exanthemas diseases; dry ears; malformation of cerumen with exfoliation of dermoid layer of meatus; **weakness**, **exhausted**, **blueness**, decomposition; alternates chill and heat; **icy cold**, **< warmth**, > cool air, chilly, thirsty.

Causticum (2)

Ringing, roaring, pulsating with deafness; words, steps re-echo; chronic middle ear catarrh; ear wax in excess; worn out; wants to die; foul smelling ear wax; **chilly**, **thirsty**.

Gelsemium (1)

Serous exudate, thin; typical flu symptoms (droopy, dizzy, weak); thirstless; may have yellow diarrhea, get giddy if too active, headache > with pressure on occiput; if take remedy and falls asleep 2–3 minutes later—correct remedy; acute necrosis of mastoid.

Hydrastis (1)

Think of with Kali mur; catarrh of middle ear, also nasopharynx—**yellow color** (Kali sulph); postnasal drip with deafness; roaring in ears; tympanic membrane bulging and purple, ears red and swollen; scabs, fissures where head connects to ear; **Eustachian catarrh** with high-pitched voice.

Kali bic (3)

Swollen; tearing pains; thick, yellow, stringy, ropy discharge; sharp stitches in left ear; thirsty; **chilly**.

Kali mur

Retracted tympanic membrane; mucus thick and white; deafness after purulent OM and from swollen Eustachian tube; swollen cervical glands; tongue coated with grey fur; feels stuffy; **chronic catarrhal conditions of middle ear**; **snapping noises in ear**, effusion around auricle.

Kali sulph

Discharge is **yellow** (Hydrastis); later stages of otitis after other remedies.

Mercurius dulcis (3)

Otitis media; Eustachian tube closed; scrofulous children; tympanic membrane retracted, thickened, immovable; deafness from every cold; > cold drinks.

Tellurium (2)

Otitis with ruptured membrane; vesicles all over; **thin**, **acrid profuse**, **long-lasting exudates which smell like pickles**; itchy, throbbing; discharge excoriates whenever it touches mucous membranes, leaves behind bleeding vesicles; severe pain deep in ear; blue-red ear with left ear <; eczema behind ear; give in low potency—does not work well in high potency.

Symptoms in Kent's Repertory	Page
Ear, Catarrah, Eustachian tube	285
Ear, Discharges, bloody/offensive	286
Ear, Discharges, purulent/thick	287
Ear, Inflammation, eustachian tube/inside	290
Ear, Inflammation, media	291
Ear, Pain, cold applications agg.	304
Ear, Pain, wrapping head amel.	306
Ear, Pain, inside/aching	307
Ear, Suppuration	318
Ear, Swelling, inside	319
Hearing, Impaired, catarrah of Eustachian tube	322

PELVIC INFLAMMATION—LEUKORRHEA

Pelvic inflammatory disease includes any inflammation of the vagina, uterus, ovaries or fallopian tubes and may involve a variety of different microorganisms. The onset may be rapid or take some time to develop and is often accompanied by intense pain, fever and chills, sweating and weakness. If allowed to go untreated, it may evolve into sepsis, perforation of the abdominal cavity, or cause sterility.

The **cause is often difficult to determine** and may appear similar to other types of abdominal inflammation such as appendicitis or irritable bowel disease. Therefore, evaluation by a physician is necessary so that the cause of the problem can be determined and treated.

Apis (3)

Itching greenish, whitish, or yellow leukorrhea, **right ovary enlarged**; lower abdominal edema, distention; **thirstless**; can crave milk; much tenderness; suppressed menses; sensation of **constriction**; labial edema > with cold water; soreness, tinging pains; dysmenorrhea with severe ovarian pain; metrorrhagia profuse with heavy abdomen, faintness; bearing-down as if menses were to appear; ovarian tumors; great tenderness over abdomen and uterus; **sudden**, **piercing cries**; profuse urine; burning urination; congestion and inflammation of **right ovary** with or without numbness down thigh; restlessness; fever.

< heat, **room**, weather
< 4 PM
< hot drinks, bed
< touch, even of hair
< after sleep
< suppressed eruptions
< right side

> cool, **air**, bathing, uncovering
> slight expectoration
> motion

Arsenicum alb (3)

Leukorrhea, acrid, excoriating, bloody, burning, copious, **instead of menses**; offensive; from standing, **thick**, white, **yellow**; burning, tensive pains in ovaries > with heat; menses profuse and too soon; pain as if from red-hot wires; **menorrhagia**; stitching pain in pelvis extending down to thigh; **sudden great weakness**; **fear**; **worry**; **restlessness**; desires sips of warm drinks; **craves ice-cold water**, which distresses stomach; **chilly**.

< cold, ices, drinks, foods	**> hot applications**; **food,** drinks
< midnight, after 2 AM	> motion; perspiring
< vegetables; **drinking**	**> elevating head**; sitting erect
< suppressed eruptions	> company
< tobacco; **exertion**	
< wet weather; seashore	
< right side	

Belladonna (3)

Right ovary; flatus from vagina; congestion of ovaries, **uterus**; swelling of uterus, **enlarged ovaries**, especially right; acute ovaritis with **throbbing pains**, < on right side; sensation of heat, congestion; comes on **suddenly**; sharp pain; bright-red, warm blood; sensation of bearing-down; breasts feel heavy; foul-smelling discharge; feels as if **all viscera would protrude at genitals**; dryness and heat of vagina; pain in sacrum, dragging in loins; **bright-red, too early and profuse menses**; cutting pain from hip to hip; diminished lochia; bearing-down > standing, < lying; back feels broken; **restlessness**; pains come and go in repeated attacks; lochia feels hot; very sensitive; slightest jarring is painful; thirsty.

< heat; afternoon (3 PM)	> light covering
< drafts, on head, haircut	> bending backward
< after taking cold	> bed rest
< check sweat; **light**; **noise**	> semi-erect
< jarring; touch; company; motion	
< hanging down	

Kreosotum (3)

Itching, **from leukorrhea**, after menses, **between labia**, **vaginal itching**, after menses; **voluptuous itching**; **leukorrhea**, morning, **acrid**, **excoriating**, bland, bloody, **burning**, copious, like menses, dark, flesh-colored, **before menses**, between menses, milky, offensive, **odor like green corn**, **putrid**, **during pregnancy**, from standing, thin, agg. walking, white, **yellow**, **stains the linen**; corrosive itching within vulva, burning and swelling of labia; **violent itching** between labia and thighs; burning and soreness in external and internal parts; bleeding after coition; menses too early, prolonged; **menstrual flow intermits** (Puls); ceases on walking or standing; reappears on lying down; pain < after menses; **intermittent** offensive lochia; leukorrhea causes holes in linen; lumpy discharges; symptoms often seen with great weakness of the legs and may be preceded by sacral or coccygeal pains; dissatisfied with everything; cross; music causes weeping; chilly.

< dentition; pregnancy	> warmth; hot food
< rest; cold; eating	> motion
< lying; summer	
< during menses	
< 6 PM to 6 AM	
< open air	
< standing & walking (leukorrhea)	> sitting (leukorrhea)

Lachesis (3)

Left ovary; voluptuous itching; leukorrhea, acrid, excoriating, copious, greenish, before menses, milky, offensive, putrid, thick, yellow; **congestion of uterus**; swelling of ovaries, uterus; uterus enlarged; begins in left ovary and moves to right; **pains relieved by the flow** (Eupion); left ovary very painful, swollen, indurated ; coccyx and sacral pain, especially on **rising** from sitting; climaxis problems; palpitations, flushes of heat; menses too short, too feeble; pain in left ovary, must lift covers off of abdomen; **loquacity**; jealousy; restless, uneasy; sensation of tension in various parts; thirsty; chilly.

< sleep, **after**, AM	**> open air**; **free discharges**
< sun	> hard pressure; bathing part

< heat, **room**, **drinks**
< swallowing, **empty**, liquids
< slightest touch of clothes
< noise; **retarded discharges**
< start and close of menses
< climaxis; **alcohol**
< cloudy weather; closing of eyes

> cold drinks; thunderstorms

Lycopodium (3)

Right ovary; itches; itches during and after menses; vaginal itching; leukorrhea, **acrid**, **excoriating**, bloody, copious, flesh-colored; **gushing**, after menses, milky, thin and watery, yellow; **swelling of ovaries**, **uterus**, vaginal dryness; menses too late, last too long, too profuse; burning of vagina from leukorrhea; discharge of blood from genitals during stool; menses with clots and serum; gas from vagina; painful coitus; **much gas**; sensitive; fearful; **fears being alone**; sensitive and grouchy in AM; chilly.

< pressure of clothes; **warmth**
< awaking; wind; right side
< eating, to satiety, oysters
< indigestion; **4–8 PM**

> warm drinks, food
> cold applications
> motion; urinating
> eructations
> after midnight

Medorrhinum (2)

From suppressed gonorrhea; itching; vaginal itching; **leukorrhea**, swelling and enlargement of ovaries, left; vaginal discharge; joint aches; restlessness, especially in legs; **offensive menses**, profuse, dark, clotted; **sensitive spot near cervical os**; thin leukorrhea, fishy odor; **sterility**; intense pruritus; frequent urination at menses; sycotic warts on genitals; ovarian pains < left side or from ovary to ovary; metrorrhagia; intense menstrual colic; many pains; fiery red, moist, violently itching anus; drawing in ovaries; > with pressure; pruritus > rubbing; hurried; nervous; restless, **time passes slowly**; weak memory.

< damp, cold; inland
< daytime; 3–4 AM
< after urinating; touch

> lying on abdomen
> bending backward; stretching
> fresh air; being fanned

< close room; before storms	> uncovering; hard rubbing
< when thinking of ailment	> seaside; sunset; dampness

Mercurius (3)

Itching, from leukorrhea, during pregnancy, **agg. by urine contact**; vaginal itching; **leukorrhea**, **night**, **acrid**, **excoriating**, bloody, copious, **in little girls**, **greenish**, lumpy, after menses, purulent, thin, white, yellow; swelling of ovaries and uterus; profuse menses with abdominal pains; **stinging ovarian pain** (Apis); itching and burning < after urination > washing with cold water; inflamed genitals, pulls at them; **easy**, **profuse sweat**; weakness, tremulous, slow in answering; breath and excretions smell foul; salivation, fever with perspiration which does not relieve; **thirsty**; chilly.

< night, night air	> moderate temperature
< sweating; **lying on right side**	
< heated; **drafts**, to head	
< changing, cloudy, cold, damp weather	
< heat and cold	
< wet feet; firelight	
< warm room, bed	

Nitric acid (3)

Itching, night, from becoming cold, **from leukorrhea**, **after menses**, **agg. walking**; **leukorrhea**, **acrid**, **excoriating**, **bloody**, **brown**, burning, copious, flesh-colored, **gonorrheal**, **greenish**, after menses, **offensive**; putrid; purulent, **ropey and stringy**, **thin**, transparent, yellow; external parts sore, with ulcers (Hep, Merc, Thuja), hair on genitals falls out (Nat m, Zinc); uterine hemorrhages; menses early, profuse, like muddy water with pain in back, hips and thighs; stitches through vagina; **splinter-like pains**; warts, large, jagged, bleed easily; cracks in skin; hateful, quarrelsome, irritable, hopeless despair; dark-complected; predominantly right side; **chilly**, thirsty.

< slight, **touch**, **jarring**, noise	> gliding motions; riding
< motion; milk; after eating	> mild weather
< cold; air; dampness	> steady pressure
< night; evening	
< weather changes; heat of bed	

< mental exertion; shock
< hot weather

Platina (2)

Itching, during menses, **voluptuous**; **leukorrhea**, morning, albuminous, bland, gonorrheal; from masturbation (Puls), before and after menses, **from sexual excitement**, **increased desire**; transparent, white; swelling of ovaries; enlarged uterus; hypersensitive genitals; tingling internally and externally (Kali brom, Orig); ovaries sensitive, burn; early menses, too profuse, **dark clotted**, with spasms and painful bearing-down, chilliness; vaginismus; nymphomania; pruritus vulvae; ovaritis with sterility; abnormal sexual appetite and melancholia; pains aggravated by pressure; violent cramping, squeezing, thrusting or numbing pains, then spasms; heat in ovaries; bruised backache > bending back; knees drawn up and spread apart; **contempt**, proud, erotic; impulse to kill; alternating mental and hysterical complaints; **cannot bear touch of clothes to genitals**; inflammation after hemorrhage.

< emotions, sexual, coition
< touch; nervous exhaustion
< sitting; standing
< evening; fasting

> walking in cool air
> sunshine

Pulsatilla (3)

Leukorrhea, **acrid**, **excoriating**, bland, **burning**, **cream-like** (Sep), in little girls, **gonorrheal**, greenish, **while lying**, **from masturbation** (Plat), before, during and after menses, **milky**, during pregnancy, from sexual excitement, thick, **thin**, **water**, white, yellow; **uterine congestion**; swelling of uterus; dry vagina; menses too late, scanty, thick, dark, **clotted**, **changeable**; **intermittent**; chilliness, nausea, downward pressure, painful flow intermits; back pains, tired feeling; **thirstless**; **weepy**, **changing symptoms**; **emotional**, **mild**.

< warmth, **air**, **room**
< getting feet wet
< suppressions; **evening**; **rest**
< beginning motion; **lying**, one side

> cold, **fresh**, **open air**
> uncovering; **erect posture**
> gentle motion; consolation; weeping
> cold food, drink

< rich foods; **fats**; ice, eggs
< puberty; **pregnancy**; before menses
< allowing feet to hang down

Sabina (3)

Inflammation after labor; itching from leukorrhea; leukorrhea, acrid, excoriating, bloody, copious, flesh-colored, gushing, jelly-like, after menses, **like boiled starch**, thick, thin, white, yellow; swelling of ovaries; enlargement of uterus; **bright red blood with pains from sacrum to pubis** or vice versa; increased sexual desire; discharge of blood between periods with sexual excitement (Ambr), **pains shoot up into vagina**; aborts easily; inflammation of uterus and ovaries after abortion; partly clotted hemorrhage **< from least motion**; **warts**, fig warts; **music is intolerable**; wants windows open.

< nightly
< heat, bed, room exercise
< pregnancy; climaxis
< foggy weather
< least motion

> cool, open air
> cold

Sepia (3)

Itching, **from leukorrhea**, during menses, **during pregnancy**, **vaginal itching**; **leukorrhea**, **morning**, **acrid**, **excoriating**, **albuminous**, bland, **bloody**, **burning**, after coition, **copious**, cream-like (Puls), flesh-colored, **in little girls**, gonorrheal, **greenish**, greenish water, **gushing**, jelly-like, lumpy, **before menses**; **between menses**, instead of menses, **milky**, **offensive**, putrid, **pregnancy**, **purulent**, thick, thin, watery, **transparent**, agg. walking; **white**, **yellow**; **congestion of uterus**; during menses; swelling of uterus; dryness of vagina; **enlarged uterus**; relaxed pelvic organs; **bearing-down sensation in pelvis, everything would escape through vulva** (Bell, Kreos, Lac c, Lil t, Nat c, Pod); **crosses limbs to prevent protrusion**; **menses too late**, **scanty**; **early and profuse**; sharp, clutching pains; violent stitches upward in vagina from uterus to umbilicus; painful vagina especially after coition; labia swollen, abscessed; angry; sensitive; irritable; averse to loved ones, sympathy; **very sad**; dreads being alone; averse to coition; chilly.

< cold, **air**, North wind, wet
< sexual excesses; abortion
< before menses; pregnancy
< morning and evening
< after first sleep; washing
< left side; after sweat
< before a thunderstorm

> violent motion; warmth
> cold drinks, bathing
> pressure; after sleep

Consider:

Aconite (3)

Ovarian inflammation; hot, dry vagina; sensitive; sharp, shooting pains; **after pains with fear**, **restlessness**; **sudden onset**.

Cantharis (3)

Puerperal metritis; with bladder inflammation; constant uterine discharge; burning ovarian pains; very sensitive; pain in coccyx, lancinating, tearing.

Cenchris

Inflammation and pain in right ovary; dark flow, dirty; cramps in right ovary.

Colocynth (1)

Cramps and spasms of uterus; **bends over double to relieve pain**; gripping pains; **burning ovarian pain**.

Lilium tig

Ovarian neuralgia; burning pains from ovary up into abdomen and down into thighs; shooting pain from left ovary across pubis or up to the breast; constant desire to support parts externally; acrid, brown leukorrhea; smarting in labia.

Origanum

Leukorrhea, **voluptuous**; sexual excesses, especially in teens.

Rhus tox (3)

Swelling, intense itching of vulva; **lochia thin**, **protracted**, **offensive**, **diminished**, **with shooting pains upward in vagina**; < first motion, > motion.

Symptoms in Kent's Repertory **Page**

Genitalia-F, Desire diminished . . . 716
Genitalia-F, Inflammation, uterus . . . 719
Genitalia-F, Itching, leukorrhea, from . . . 720
Genitalia-F, Leukorrhea, acrid, excoriating/burning . . . 721
Genitalia-F, Leukorrhea, menses, before . . . 722
Genitalia-F, Pain, uterus . . . 733
Genitalia-F, Pain, vagina, coition, after . . . 734
Genitalia-F, Sensitive, vagina . . . 744
Genitalia-F, Swollen . . . 744

PNEUMONIA—BRONCHIAL LOBAR

Pneumonia is caused by an infection of the lung tissue by either a bacteria or virus. Symptoms include fever and chills, shortness of breath accompanied by a productive cough with expectoration of a yellowish to greenish to blood-stained mucus. Additionally there may be sweating, lethargy and prostration.

In general, **bacterial pneumonia** results in a higher fever and is considered more severe than its **viral** counterpart. While it is seen more commonly in **children** and the **elderly**, these age groups may not exhibit the usual signs and symptoms of the disease, which can lead to its being missed. If untreated or incompletely treated, pneumonia can spread quickly throughout the lungs, causing severe respiratory difficulties and death. Since the course of the disease can progress very rapidly, evaluation by a physician is most important.

Aconite (3)

Inflammation of lungs; left lung; in infants; **pleural pneumonia**; constant pressure in left chest; **oppression of breathing** on least motion; **hoarse**, **dry**, **croupy cough**; loud, labored breathing; sensitive to inspired air; short of breath; cough **< at night**, **after midnight**; hot feeling in lungs; bloody sputum; chest tingles after cough; stitching pain in chest; **burning thirst**; **anxious**; **fearful**; **high fever**; perspiration, may or may not relieve; sudden, violent onset; cold sweat; **cold passes through in waves**; dry heat, red face; cold and heat alternate.

< sleeping in sun; warm room
< fright; **shock**
< cold, dry winds; perspiring
< pressure, touch; tobacco smoke
< noise; light; dentition
< menses; night; lying on side

> open air; repose
> warm sweat

Antimonium tart (3)

Inflammation of lungs; in infants; **pleura-pneumonia**; rheumatic pleural pneumonia; **much rattling of mucus in chest but little expectoration**; velvety feeling in chest, burning sensation rising to throat; rapid, short breaths, feel as if they will **suffocate**, sits up; **coughing and gasping consecutively**; **edema and impending paralysis of lungs**; pulse rapid, weak, trembling; cough and dyspnea > lying on right side (opposite Badiaga); sensation as if a crushing weight on chest; coughs and yawns alternately; coldness, trembling, chilliness, **copious**; sticky perspiration; **lack of reaction**; peevish, whining; fear of being alone; despondent; paleness of face; sunken.

< warm, room, weather, wraps
< anger; lying; morning
< overeating; cold; dampness
< evening; sour things; milk

> expectoration; vomiting
> sitting erect; motion

Arsenicum alb (3)

Inflammation of lungs; pleura; **neglected pleural pneumonias**; expectoration is rust-colored; blood-streaked, pink; unable to lie down for fear of suffocation; burning of chest; cough < lying on back; after midnight; **darting pain through upper third of right lung**; wheezing respiration; burning heat all over; dry cough; rapid pulse; dry tongue; **intermittent**, septic fevers; cold sweats; intense heat about 3 AM; **very restless**; **periodicity marked with adynamia**; **putrid cadaveric odor**; **burning thirst craves ice cold drinks**; **or sips of warm drinks**; **nightly aggravations**; pulmonary edema; frothy expectoration; **cold** externally with burning heat internal; **chilly**, **thirsty**; **fears death**; **must move constantly**; burning > with heat; oliguria.

< cold, **ices**, **drinks**, **foods**
< cold air
< after midnight; 2 AM
< vegetables; **drinking**
< eruptions, suppressed, undeveloped
< lying on part; tobacco, **exertion**

> hot, **applications**, **food**, drink
> motion; **elevating head**
> company; sitting erect
> perspiration

< wet weather; right side
< seashore

Bryonia (3)

Inflammation lungs; **right lung**; elderly, in infants; **pleura pneumonia**, right, **rheumatic**; stitching pain < right side; **> lying on painful side**; dry tongue; intense heat; dry cough with fever; cough at night, **must sit up**; **< eating or drinking**; expectorates blood or rust-colored mucus; difficult, quick respiration, with frequent desire to take a long breath; **must support chest when coughing**; thick, tough mucus in trachea; **coming into warm room causes cough** (Nat c); heavy sensation beneath sternum extends toward right shoulder; **pulse full**, **hard**, **tense**, **quick**; chilled with external coldness; internal heat; sour sweat after slight exertion; easy, profuse perspiration; dry, friction sound on auscultation; pleurisy; **averse to motion**; **bursting headaches**; **irritable**; delirious; **dryness of mucous membranes**; **thirst**; **for large quantities**.

< motion; **rising**; **stooping**
< dry, heat & cold
< deep breathing
< becoming warm; **warm room**; weather
< drinking while hot; **eating**
< vexation; light touch
< suppressions; taking cold
< early AM; **cough**

> pressure; **lying on painful part**
> cool open air; **quiet**
> cloudy, damp days
> drawing knees up
> heat to inflamed part
> rest

Ferrum phos (3)

Inflammation of lungs; in infants, pleural pneumonia; **early stages of febrile conditions**; congestion of lungs; bloody sputum; short, painful, tickling cough; hard, dry cough with sore chest; **expectoration of pure blood in pneumonia** (Mill); cough > at night; rapid, **short**, **quick**, **soft pulse**; bruised soreness; chest heavy; sore; congested; perspiration; heat with sweaty hands; thirsty.

< night (4–6 AM); motion
< noise; jarring; cold air
< checked sweat; right side

> cold; application
> lying down; bleeding

Kali carb (2)

Inflammation of lungs, right lung, **right lower lobe**; infants; aggravated lying on right side; after measles; pleural pneumonia; cutting chest pains; dry, hard cough, about 3 AM: **stitching pains** and dryness of pharynx; **whole chest very sensitive**; scanty, thick expectoration which **increases** in AM and after eating; leaning forward relieves chest symptoms; **coldness of chest**; **wheezing**; lungs seem to stick to ribs; pleurisy; chest pains toward left scapula; pulse small, soft, variable, intermittent, **chilly**; with hot hands; never wants to be left alone; **perspiration**, **weakness**, **backache**; **intolerance of cold**; **hypersensitive** to pain; **irritable**; discontented; thirsty; mucus purulent, blood-streaked; yellow face; respiration < with heat.

< cold, **air**, water, drafts	> warmth; sitting with elbows on knees
< after overheating; exertion	> open air; movement
< 2–3 AM; winter; before menses	> daytime
< lying on painful or left side	
< fluid loss; soup; coffee	

Lycopodium (3)

Inflammation of lungs, right lung, in infants; **neglected pneumonias**; stitching pains on right side; thoracic pain < respiration; rusty, purulent, blood-streaked sputum; flaring nostrils; dyspnea; cough is deep, hollow, **salty** expectoration (Ars, Phos, Puls, Sep), chest seems full of rattling mucus; fever with chilling, especially 3–4 AM followed by sweat; icy coldness, patient feels as if lying on ice; one chill followed by another; repeating or alternating symptoms; **much gas**; rapid pulse; burning between scapulae; chilly; **perspiration**; intolerance of cold drinks; **craves warmth**; **fear of being alone**; **apprehensive**; headstrong and haughty when sick.

< pressure of clothes; **warmth**	**> warm drinks**, food
< awaking; wind; **4–8 PM**	> cold applications; **motion**
< eating; to satiety; oysters	> eructations; urinating
< right side; from right to left	> after midnight
< from above to down	> being uncovered
< warm applications except to throat	

Mercurius (3)

Inflammation of lung; right lung; right lower lobe; in infants; pleural pneumonia; cough, with yellow mucopurulent sputum; **cannot lie on right side** (left Lyc); catarrh, with chilliness; dread of air; stitches from lower lobe to right lung to back; **profuse** nightly **perspiration**; debility from perspiration; heat and shuddering alternately; **creeping chilliness** < evening, night; **much saliva**; **metallic taste**; respiration < lying on left side but cough < lying on right; perspiration does not relieve; debility; mistrustful; weary; **intense thirst for cold drinks**; chilly.

< night; air; **heated**	> moderate temperatures
< sweating; **lying on right side**	
< sensitive; **drafts**, to head	
< weather changes; cloudy	
< taking cold; temperature extremes	
< wet feet; firelight	
< warm room; bed	

Phosphorus (3)

Inflammation of lungs, right lung, right lower lobe, left lung, in infants; lies on back with head thrown back; lying on back ameliorates; **pleural pneumonia**; rusty, purulent, blood-streaked sputum; stitching chest pains; hard, dry, tight, racking cough, **< cold air**; cough from warm room into cold air; burning; **heat** in chest; **increased**, **oppressed respiration**, **tightness across chest**, **weight on chest**; pneumonia **< lying on left side**; whole body **trembles** with cough; respiratory difficulties with the heat; chilly every evening; **adynamic with lack of thirst**, unnatural hunger; viscid night sweats; profuse perspiration; **craves cold drinks**; listless; **apathetic**; **indifferent**; anxious, from being alone; **chilly**.

< lying on left side, **back**	> eating; sleeping
< emotions; slightest talking, touch odors, light	> cold, food, water to face
< cold, **hands** in water, open air	> rubbing
< lying on painful side	> sitting up; in dark
< salt; puberty; sexual excesses	> lying on right side

< weather; changes; thunderstorms, windy
< AM, PM; mental fatigue

Senega (3)

Inflammation of lungs, in elderly, **pleural pneumonia**, neglected pleural pneumonia; bursting pain in back after cough; circumscribed spots in chest after inflammation; thorax feels too narrow; **cough often ends in a sneeze**; **rattling in chest** (Ant t); oppression in chest on ascending; bronchial catarrh **with sore chest walls**; sensation of oppression, weight on chest; **difficulty in raising tough**, **profuse mucus**, in aged; old asthmatics with congestion; **pleural exudates**; hydrothorax (Merc, Sulph); pressure on chest as if lungs forced back to spine, burning of air passages; subacute states; blood-stained or albuminous expectoration; pains shift on stooping.

< air, open, wind, inhaling cold	> motion; in open air
< rest; pressure; touch	**> bending head back**
< looking fixedly	> sweating

Sulphur (3)

Inflammation of lungs, left lung, left lower lobe, must lie on back, lying on back ameliorates, **neglected pneumonias**, **pleural pneumonia**, rheumatic mucopurulent, bloody, expectoration; oppression and burning in chest; **difficult respiration**; **wants windows open**; heat in chest; red, brown spots all over chest; loose cough < talking, morning; greenish, sweetish sputum; **much rattling in chest**; chest feels heavy, with heart feeling too large, palpitating; stitching pains shoot through to back, < lying on back or breathing deeply; **dyspnea in middle of night**, **> sitting up**; **pulse more rapid in AM than PM**, **suffocative air hunger**; irregular breathing; chest pain backward from left nipple; rattling and heat in chest at 11 AM: **frequent flushes of heat**; dry skin, great thirst; night sweats, nape of neck and occiput; forgetful, **selfish**, peevish, delusions; irritable; **thirsty**; chilly; consider Lycopodium to follow.

< suppressions, **bathing**; milk	> open air; motion
< heated; **exertion**; **in bed**	> warm applications
< atmospheric changes; speaking	> sweating; dry heat
< 11 AM; full moon; periodically	> drawing up affected limbs

< rest; standing
< alcohol

Consider:

Calcarea carb (2)

Inflammation of lungs; upper lobes, left lobe, pleural pneumonia; neglected pneumonias; painless hoarseness; chest very sensitive to touch (Lach); pressure, percussion; tight, burning, sore chest, < going up stairs; extreme dyspnea.

Carbo veg (3)

Inflammation of lungs, pleural pneumonia, wheezing, rattling of mucus in chest; **cough with burning in chest**; **must be fanned**; lung hemorrhages; coldness with thirst; exhausting sweats.

Chelidonium (3)

Inflammation of lungs, right upper lobe; left lower lobe; quick, short respirations; pain in right side of chest and shoulder; loose rattling with difficult expectoration; **pain under inner and lower right scapula**.

Ipecac (2)

Inflammation of chest **in infants**; **cough incessant**, **violent with every breath**; chest full of phlegm but does not expectorate; bubbling rales; child becomes stiff, blue in face; **constriction in chest**; **slightest chill with much heat**, **nausea** and vomiting; coughs; vomits.

Lobelia (3)

Inflammation of lungs; in infants; **dyspnea from constriction in chest**; sensation of pressure or weight on chest; < any exertion.

Pulsatilla (3)

Inflammation of lungs, dry cough evening and night; **must sit up to get relief, cough is loose in AM**; **pressure on chest**; **soreness**; short breath, anxiety; palpitations when lying on left side; **chilliness**, even in a warm room; **without thirst**; intolerable burning heat at night; **thirstless**; **> open air**.

Rhus tox (3)

Inflammation of lungs, pleura pneumonia; **dry**, **teasing cough**, from midnight until AM, **during chill or when putting hands out of bed**; hemoptysis, bright red; oppression of chest, sticking pains; intermittent fevers, dryness; chilly as if cold water poured over them followed by heat and inclination to stretch limbs.

Sepia (3)

Inflammation of lungs, neglected pneumonias; oppression of chest AM, PM: cough in AM, with profuse expectoration, tastes salty (Ars, Lyc, Phos, Puls); frequent flushes of heat; sweat from least motion; shivering with thirst; chilly.

Silicea (2)

Slow recovery after pneumonia; **neglected pneumonias**; **violent cough when lying down with thick**, **yellow**, **lumpy sputum**; chilly, very sensitive to cold air; cold extremities; even in a warm room; sweat at night, < towards morning.

Veratrum viride (3)

Inflammation of lungs; difficult respiration; sensation of a heavy load on chest; pneumonia with faint feeling in stomach and violent congestion; increased fever in evening; decreased in AM.

Symptoms in Kent's Repertory	**Page**
Respiration, Difficult, lying, while	769
Cough, see various times	778
Cough, Deep	783
Cough, Rattling	801
Cough, Sitting Up, must	803
Expectoration, Mucous, bloody	817
Expectoration, Purulent	817
Chest, Abscess, lung	822
Chest, Hepatization of lungs	834
Chest, Inflammation, lungs	835

POISONING, FOOD

Reactions to water or foods tainted with fungal or bacterial overgrowth and toxins will vary among individuals and are dependent upon the amount of contaminated material present and the quantity of food or water ingested. Signs and symptoms of **food poisoning** usually begin to occur several hours after eating or drinking and may have a gradual onset, which builds in intensity as the toxins are absorbed.

Generally, the person complains of nausea and stomach pains or cramping which may range from mild to severe. There is often a feeling of weakness which may get progressively worse, or outright prostration. Vomiting and/or diarrhea usually accompany the condition as the body attempts to eliminate the toxic materials. Fever is not uncommon as the body attempts to burn off the excess wastes. There may also be an accompanying skin rash otherwise known as urticaria, which appears as large red splotches.

In some cases, the progression may be so rapid as to precipitate a **shock-like condition**. The person should be evaluated by a physician but can be given charcoal capsules which absorb the toxic materials and counteract the diarrhea until they can be seen.

Agaricus

Symptoms occur several hours (3 to 12) after ingestion of food; stomach is distended, rumbling, with flatulence; burning in the stomach begins about 3 hours after eating then changes to a dull pressure; **gastric upset with sharp pains in region of the liver and spleen**; empty eructations which may taste like rotten eggs, apples; sensation of an **icy coldness which feels like needles**, over various parts of the body; from alcohol poisoning, with delirium (Bell); may have double vision, blurred vision (Gels); diarrhea with flatus, nausea; very sensitive to touch; may have a loss of muscular control.

< alcohol
< cold, cold air

Arsenicum alb

Stomach upset, **burning pains** from **food** or drink (Phos); heartburn, following eructations of acid and bile from the stomach, continued belching and eructations; **poisoning from contaminated water**; aggravated **by vegetables**, **fruits**, **melons**; **nausea**, from smell of food (Colch, Sep); **diarrhea**, with **burning** in the rectum; **vomiting**, **of blood**, bile; burning in the stomach, > milk; patient may want **cold water** to drink, **which is vomited immediately** (Phos) or **warm drinks** which are taken in sips; stomach pains < cold food, drink, > external heat and warm drinks; stomach is very sensitive to touch (Nux v); patient is **weak**, **prostrated** and mentally or physically **restless**; **chilly**; **thirsty**.

< cold drinks	> external heat
< night	> warm drinks

Carbo veg

Excessive **belching** following eating or drinking, which relieves temporarily; eructations which are sour, putrid; burning stomach pains which extend to the back, **contractive pain which extends to chest**, **accompanied by distention of the abdomen**; cramping in stomach causes the patient to bend double (Coloc); epigastric region sensitive to touch, tight things around waist (Lach, Nux v); **sense of heaviness**, **fullness** in abdomen, especially the upper part, is > with passing flatus; belching may or may not relieve; **slow digestion** with subsequent **putrification**; nausea in AM (Sep), patient may be adverse to milk, meat, **fatty foods** (Puls), but craves coffee, sweets, salt and acid things; condition causes the person to be weak; **chilly**; thirsty, which isn't > with drinking; stools are loose, dysenteric-like, hot, foul-smelling; may have **coldness**, **blueness of the skin** and a **desire to be fanned**, **for fresh air**.

< depletions	> eructations
< rich foods, alcohol	**> cool air**, **being fanned**
< pressure, of clothes	
< evenings; warmth	

Cuprum ars

Nausea and vomiting which is < after eating; nausea from burning and a distressed feeling in the upper abdomen; burning pains may run from mouth to stomach; **violent cramping pains** in the bowels with rectal and vesicle tenesmus; sharp, shooting abdominal pains; increased cramping and rumbling in abdomen, followed by a profuse diarrhea which is a slimy, dark liquid; **cramping of legs**, **arms**; moderate thirst, but drinking causes an increase in the nausea; good remedy for cholera (Ars, Camph, Verat), typhoid, **uremic poisoning**; **urine** may have a **garlicky odor** to it; (consider Cupr met and Arsenicum alb).

< pressure, touch

Ferrum met—See Gastritis.

Ipecac—See Nausea and Vomiting of Pregnancy.

Nux vomica—See Gastritis.

Veratrum album—See Gastritis.

Urtica urens

Shellfish poisoning, especially if there is **urticaria** with **intense itching** and red blotches with burning and stinging pains, which are < with cold (opp Apis), and may be > with warmth; edema; soreness of abdomen, < lying down; stitching pains in region of the spleen; slimy stools.

< lying down

Consider:

Botulinum

Nosode of botulinum bacillus toxin; **food poisoning**, **canned**; cramping in the stomach; staggering, dizziness and a slurring or thickening of speech; blurred or double vision, ptosis of the eyelids (Gels); difficulty with swallowing, choking sensation and may have difficulty breathing.

Pyrogenum

If sepsis occurs.

Symptoms in Kent's Repertory **Page**

PROSTATITIS—PROSTATIC ENLARGEMENT

By the age of 50, about 30% of all men will experience difficulties with urination that are related to **enlargement** or **inflammation** of the **prostate gland**. Between the ages of 20 and 50, problems with the prostate usually are associated with infection known as prostatitis. This may include symptoms of high fever, chills, a sense of fatigue, and frequent and painful urination. **Prostatitis** may become a chronic condition, resulting in burning on urination, frequency of urination and a mild but irritating perineal pain. There may also be no symptoms present at all and the person may have had the infection for many years.

Prostatitis is associated with infection by a variety of organisms and often accompanies increased amounts of sexual activity, especially if there are multiple partners. Infection which is untreated or unrecognized can result in reinfection of the partner. If allowed to continue, the condition can lead to a systemic bacterial infection or possibly sterility as it spreads to the rest of the genital urinary tract.

Apis (3)

Emission of prostatic fluid; enlarged; **inflammation**; painful during urination; pressing sensation; burning soreness during urination; frequent and involuntary; incontinence; **last drops burn**; cannot urinate without a stool; **scanty**, **colored urine**; **constricted** sensations; edema; sharp **stinging**; sudden cries of pain; thirstless.

< heat, **room**, weather, drinks	**> cool**, **air**, bathing
< heat, bed, water	> uncovering; motion
< touch, even of hair	> slight expectoration
< after sleep; 4 PM	
< pressure; suppressed eruptions	
< right side	

Baryta carb (3)

Enlarged prostate, **especially in elderly**; diminished desire; premature impotence; induration of testicles; urging; burning in urethra with urination; protrusion of piles with urination; senile dementia; loss of memory; numbness of genitals; **slow**; erections with riding; thirsty, **chilly**.

< company; cold, damp
< cold to feet, to head
< lying on painful side
< left side; odors; washing
< thinking of symptoms

> warm wraps
> walking in open air

Berberis (2)

Enlarged prostate; painful; pressing pains; smarting, burning, stitching in testicles, prepuce and scrotum; **pain in thighs and loins on urinating**; frequent urination; urethra burns when not urinating; **thick mucus and bright red urine** passed; sensation as if some urine remains after urinating; pains **radiating** from one spot; many rapidly changing symptoms; **gurgling** or bubbling; urinary calculi; thirsty; standing brings on or increases urinary complaint.

< motion; jarring; rising and sitting
< fatigue; urinating
< standing

Calcarea carb (3)

Enlargement of prostate; emission of prostatic fluid, with stool, after stool, after urination; **frequent emissions**; increased desire; premature ejaculation; weakness after coition; enuresis; irritable bladder; crawling, constriction in rectum; foul or strong odor of urine; hydrocele; **thirsty**; **chilly**.

< cold, **air**, wet, **bathing**
< weather changes; standing
< exertion, mental, physical, ascending
< pressure of clothes; **milk**
< anxiety; awaking; water
< full moon

> dry climate, weather
> lying on painful side

Chimaphila (3)

Inflammation of prostate; enlarged prostate, emission of prostatic fluid; painful, while sitting, pressing pain, **soreness**; **swelling of prostate**; **scanty urine with much ropy**, **mucopurulent sediment**; smarting in urethra from neck of bladder to meatus; urging; burning, scalding during urination; straining after urination; must strain before flow comes; acute prostatitis, retention and **feeling of a ball in perineum** (Cann i); unable to urinate without feet wide apart and body inclined forward, **sugar in urine**; good remedy for urethritis and prostatitis.

< cold, damp	> walking
< standing; sitting	
< beginning urination	
< sitting on cold	
< left side	

Conium (3)

Enlarged prostate, **hardness**; emission of prostatic fluid, **with emotions**, without erections, with passing flatus, **during lascivious thoughts**, **with stool**, difficult stool; **heaviness sensation**; induration; inflammation; pain, biting, pressing, stitching; swelling; increased desire but decreased power; testis hard, enlarged; **effects of suppressed sexual appetite**; much difficulty voiding; **flows then stops then flows** (Ledum); **debility**; **stony hardness**; cutting sensation with ejaculation; depressed, **interrupted discharge** (Clematis); acute cutting pains felt in neck of bladder with shooting pain in the orifice; thirsty; chilly.

< seeing objects moving	> letting part hang down
< alcohol; raising arms	> fasting; in the dark
< after erections; injury	> motion; pressure
< night; sexual excesses	
< cold; old age; **celibacy**	
< lying; with head low	
< turning or rising in bed	

Digitalis (3)

Enlarged prostate, in elderly; inflammation, from suppressed gonorrhea; feeling of irritation; painful, while sitting, while straining with urinating; swelling; nightly emissions, with weakness of genitals after coitus; hydrocele, enlarged scrotum; urging; urine in drops, dark, hot, burning with **throbbing** pain at neck of bladder, **as if a straw were being thrust back and forth**; full feeling after urination; **urethritis**; constriction and burning as if urethra were to small; early AM erections; balanitis (Merc); chilly, **thirsty**, **anxiety** about future, despondent.

Lycopodium (2)

Emission of prostatic fluid (Agn, Calad, Sel), without erections; enlarged prostate; inflammation; pain, pressing, during urination, stitching; **impotence**; premature emissions; pain in back before urination, ceases after flow; **urine slow in coming**, must strain; frequent urging > riding; scanty urine, cries before passing it; **much flatulence**; chilly.

< pressure of clothes; **warmth**
< awaking; wind; eating
< indigestion; **4–8 PM**
< right side; right to left
< warm applications

> warm drinks, food
> cold applications; motion
> eructations; urinating

Medorrhinum (2)

Enlarged prostate; hardness of prostate; inflammation; swelling; painful tenesmus with urinating; **nocturnal enuresis**; urine flows slowly; **impotence**; frequent and painful urination; sensation of heaviness in lower abdomen or prostate; chilly; nervous; restless, **time passes slowly**.

< damp, cold
< daytime; 3–4 AM
< after urinating; touch
< closed room; before storms
< thinking of ailments
< heat

> lying on abdomen
> bending backward; stretching
> fresh air; being fanned
> uncovering; hard pressure
> seaside; sunset; dampness

Pareira brava (2)

Enlarged prostate; inflammation; pain, during urination, stitching during urination; sensation as if bladder distended, with pain (Staph); **pain travels down thigh**; **constant urging**; **great straining**; dribbling; **violent pain in glans**; itching of urethra; can emit urine only with being on his knees pressing head firmly against floor; black, bloody urine; thick mucus; left side; dribbling after urination (Sel).

> on hands and knees

Pulsatilla (3)

Enlargement of prostate; emission of prostatic fluid, with emotions; during erections; **inflammation**, from suppressed gonorrhea; pain, **after urination**, constrictive, pressing, stitching; swelling; pain from abdomen to testicles, stricture; urine passes only in drops, interrupted stream; **acute prostatitis**; pain and tenesmus with urinating, **< lying on back**; increased desire; **< with lying down**; involuntary passing of urine with cough, passing flatus; spasmodic pain in bladder after urinating; **thick**, **yellow-green discharges**; **shifting symptoms**, sensation as if a stone is rolling down bladder; nocturnal enuresis; **thirstless**, **desires fresh air**; more often useful in orchitis.

< warmth, **air**, **room**
< getting feet wet
< suppressions; **evening**
< rest
< rich foods; **eating**; **fats**, ices
< on painless side; allowing feet to hang down

> cold, **fresh**, **open air**
> uncovering; **erect posture**
> gentle motion; continued motion
> weeping

Sabal serrulata (1)

Emission of prostatic fluid; inflammation; chronic or acute enlargements, with difficulty passing urine; burning with urination; wasting of testis; **loss of sexual power**; coitus painful at times of emission; organs feel cold; **sexual neurotics**; sharp, stinging pains in urethra; enuresis; painful erections; backache from coition; **fear of going to sleep**; **epididymitis**; **enuresis**.

< old men
< weather, cold, damp, cloudy
< sympathy

Selenium (2)

Emission of prostatic fluid, with emotions, while sitting, **with stool**, soft stool, after stool, **after urination**; enlarged, **in elderly**; induration; inflammation; pain, pressing, stitching during urination; swelling; sensation in tip of urethra as if a biting drop were forcing its way out; involuntary dribbling, urine, prostatic fluid; **loss of sexual power**, with lascivious fancies; **increased desire**; **decreased power**; relaxation of penis with coitus; **hydrocele**; exertion makes him sleepy; loquacity.

< hot days; sexual excesses
< loss of sleep; singing
< drafts; after sleep
< tea; lemonade
< heat

> after sunset
> inhaling cool air

Thuja (2)

Enlargement; emission of prostatic fluid; **induration**; inflammation, from suppressed gonorrhea; pain, aching during urination, pressing; swelling; tension; acute inflammation from gonorrhea; chronic induration of testis; **gonorrhea**; frequent and urgent desire to urinate with pain and burning felt at neck of bladder; urinary stream is split, small; sensation of trickling after urination or severe cutting (Sars); sudden desire and urgency to urinate, cannot be controlled; paralysis of sphincter; profuse sweat on genitals; wandering pains; warts; thirsty; chilly.

< cold, damp
< heat, of bed; at night
< 3 AM & 3 PM: increasing moon
< urinating; vaccination
< tea; onions; fat; coffee

> warm, wind, air
> wrapping head
> free secretions; sneezing
> motion; touch
> crossing legs; left side
> drawing up a limb

Consider:

Benzoic acid (2)

Swelling right side of testis; profuse urination; enlarged prostate; **strong odor of urine**.

Cannabis indica

Sensation of a ball in anal region; **backache after coitus**; dribbling of urine; **strains to urinate**.

Clematis (1)

Enlarged prostate; **interrupted flow**, constricted urethra; urine emitted drop by drop, swelling and induration of testis, **bruised feeling**.

Iodum (2)

Enlarged prostate; induration; swollen and indurated or emaciated testis; loss of sexual power; frequent urination.

Nitric acid (2)

Enlarged prostate; inflammation; **from suppressed gonorrhea**; soreness, burning, stitching pains; profuse urine in old prostatic cases.

Silicea (2)

Suppuration of prostate; prostatic fluid discharge with straining at stool; burning and soreness of genitals, with eruption on inner surface of thighs; **ill effects of vaccination**.

Spongia (2)

Enlargement; **swelling of spermatic cord and testis with pain, tenderness, orchitis**.

Staphysagria (2)

Enlargement; inflammation; **sensation as if a drop of urine were rolling continuously along urethra**, frequent urination; **burning when not urinating in urethra**; **emission of prostatic fluid**.

Sulphur (2)

Enlargement; inflammation; involuntary emissions of urine; **sudden urgency**.

Symptoms in Kent's Repertory **Page**

Bladder, Retention, enlarged prostate.................. 651
Prostate Gland, Enlargement.......................... 667
Prostate Gland, Inflammation, gonorrhea............... 668
Urethra, Agglutination of meatus...................... 669
Urethra, Discharge, bloody/gleety...................... 669
Urethra, Discharge, gonorrheal/greenish............... 670
Urethra, Inflammation, meatus......................... 672
Urethra, Itching, gonorrhea/fossa navicularis........... 672
Urethra, Pain, urination during........................ 673
Urethra, Pain, burning, urination, before............... 674
Urethra, Stricture..................................... 679
Genitalia, Seminal discharge, bloody/painful........... 709

See **Urethritis**

SHOCK/COLLAPSE

Shock is a condition that is considered a **medical emergency** and needs prompt attention, as time is of the essence. While the events leading up to shock and collapse may be varied, once the chain of events has begun, any means necessary to reverse the condition must be used in order to prevent brain damage or suffocation and death. The cause (e.g. trauma, drowning, heat stroke, etc.) should be determined if possible, as it will help with remedy selection as well as management of the patient.

The person may appear pale and exhibit a weak pulse and shallow breathing, or be bluish in color from lack of oxygen. **Knowledge of CPR procedures** is valuable and often needed, as immediate assessment of the person's pulse and respiratory status are imperative. The person should be kept warm and dry and comfortable as possible. Someone should be sent for help while the person is being assisted.

Even with successful homeopathic treatment, the person needs to be further evaluated by a physician to determine if there has been any permanent damage suffered.

Aconite (3)

Fear, fright and anxiety characterize the state just before or with collapse; **sudden, violent** onset; **tingling coldness** and **numbness** of the body; delirium with **fear, worry** and **restlessness** but unconsciousness is not often seen; may have vertigo which is < rising (Nux v, Op); face may be red, hot, flushed or swollen which **becomes deathly pale with sitting up**, with **dizziness**, difficult to lie on side but is < lying on back; may have **vomiting from the fear**; **oppressed breathing, < motion**, short of breath and patient is very **sensitive to cold air** (Hep, Nux v; opp. Camph, Carbo veg); may have increased heart rate with **palpitations** and a **full, hard, intense** pulse; sensation of **cold waves** or water **passing through them** (Verat a) with the fever and is accompanied **by thirst** and **restlessness**; **anxiety** and a **fear of death** may be prominent.

< touch, pressure
< cold, cold air
< motion

> perspiration

Arnica (3)

Shock from injuries, **blows**, **falls**, especially those to the head; consider as a first remedy if condition came on after some type of injury or vascular lesion such as thrombosis or hemorrhage; unconsciousness, confused drowsiness, will answer questions correctly but then relapse; as the condition becomes worse, the patients may try to express themselves but are unable to, will misjudge the situation and underestimate its severity, may wish to be left alone and **tell you that help is not needed** (Ars, Bapt, Carb v); patient may complain of bed being too hard even though it is soft; may have a loss of sphincter control during the stupor; **head is hot**, **with a coldness of the body**, **sunken face** which is very red; drowsiness with yawning (Nux m); **very weak** which may lead to faintness, from the **heat of the sun**, **motion**; may have a feeling they are going to die.

< motion; touch
< cold, cold damp

> lying down
> lying with head low

Camphor (3)

Collapse, **with icy coldness** (Ars, Carbo v) **of whole body**; very sudden weakness with a weak pulse; pupils dilated and/or fixed, with staring; ***patient does not want to be covered even though they are icy cold;*** may froth at the mouth, blueness of the lips; lockjaw (Lyssin); may have a sensation of **internal burning** and **heat**; very **anxious**, sense of impending death (Acon, Ars); **insensible**, with loss of memory; cramping in extremities with coldness, numbness and tingling; **does not want to be alone** (Ars); eyes sunken, pupils contracted and eyes turned upward (Op); head pain ***which is > by thinking about it,*** may also apply to other pains; blood shunts to interior causing skin to be cold, pale, blue, with a drop in blood pressure; excellent medicine for lockjaw, cholera.

< cold, open air
< night; motion

> warmth
> thinking of pains

Carbo veg (2)

Stagnation of the blood with an **icy coldness** (Ars, Camph), **blueness** of skin and **ecchymosis from sluggishness of blood flow**; after loss of fluids; patient appears lifeless, but may have a hot head, cool breath and a very weak pulse, **desires to be fanned**, **wants windows open**, **air to flow on them**; face is puffy, cyanotic, cold with cold perspiration, may be blue with red splotches, especially if patient drinks coffee, alcohol; twitching of facial muscles, especially the **upper lip**; paleness of the face; head feels heavy, painful; watery blisters may form on the lips; lack of vital reaction, difficult to arouse (Op); **burning pains internally with being cold externally**; may have oozing of blood from mucus membranes, old injuries, which tend to ulcerate; confusion, difficulty with thinking, very indifferent; may be anxious and restless, especially at night; pulse is weak, intermittent, thread-like; may have heart palpitations; patient may feel a pulsation which spreads upward; patient **wants to drink cold water during the chills**; very exhausting night and morning sweats may occur; thirsty for cold water; good medicine for cholera (Camphor, Verat a), typhoid, sepsis.

< becoming cold
< loss of fluids
< warm, damp

> being fanned
> cool air

Opium (3)

Insensibility, especially of the nerves, **painlessness**; **drowsy**, **stupor**; intense **sleepiness** (Nux m); **sluggishness of function**, lack of vital reaction (Carb v); **placid**, convulsions or shock **following fear or fright** and may have been preceded by an excited state; pupils contracted (Camph), dilated, **insensible to light**, eyes half-closed and or upturned; muscles of the face twitch, tremble; **face is sweaty**, red, hot or pale, may alternate between redness and paleness; lower jaw drops, may have bloody frothing from the mouth, difficulty speaking, swallowing; face may be cyanotic or purple in color; pulse is weak, **very slow**; there is an overall absence of sensations, painlessness and paralysis of functional activity; respiration is **irregular**, slow and may stop for a period of time before starting again (Cheyne-Stokes); thirsty.

< alcohol	> caffeine, coffee
< heat	> cold air
< fear, **fright**	> walking
	> physical stimulation

Veratrum alb (3)

Collapse with **extreme coldness and blueness of parts**, with **weakness**; good for shock following surgery; patient has **cold sweat on forehead**, rapid and fibulae pulse with a pale face; may be alternately manic and in a stupor; unresponsive to external stimuli (Op); **sudden** and **violent onset of condition** (Acon); fainting from emotions, exertion, injuries and from hemorrhages; person is **very cold** as is their breath; **delirium** with violence, lewdness and loquacity, especially with the pains; face is pale, **bluish**, distorted, cold and may have a terrified look, face is flushed with lying but breaks out in a cold sweat with getting up, **especially on the forehead**; loss of vision may occur; vertigo; headache with nausea and vomiting, head may feel alternately hot and cold with heaviness, numbness and confused mentation; there may be a sensation as if ice has been applied to the top of the head or a cold wind or water has been poured on it; patient may be restless but movement causes further prostration and weakness; collapse from intense vomiting and purging, with extreme coldness and weakness, as in cholera (Camphor, Cupr); thirsty.

< motion; fright	> uncovering; night
< heat	> warmth
< cold drinks	

Consider:

Cuprum met (2)

Consider if preceded by **convulsions** or **epileptic fits**; patient is exhausted, shivering, shows poor reaction to stimulation and is confused; face is **blue**, pale, distorted and may have a **chewing motion of the lower jaw**; eyes are fixed, staring and may be turned upward or rolling; **cramping** of **muscles**; consider if onset is after suppressed eruptions; see under convulsions.

Gelsemium (2)

Confusion, apathy, **dazed**, **weakness**; patient is **drowsy**, **droopy and dull**, condition often follows fear, fright or anxiety; **dilated pupils** with **heavy** and **drooping eyelids**; **extreme weakness**; dropping of lower jaw; patient wants to sleep; thirstless; see under **heat stroke**.

Nux moschata

Sleepiness, **dreamy state**, **drowsy**, bewildered, thinks they are in a dream, slow to think and a vanishing of thought; head drops forward with sitting and may feel sick with rising up from lying; face is pale, jaw may seem as if it is paralyzed; **extreme dryness of the mucous membranes**; **complaints cause sleepiness**, **coma**; **yet thirstless** (Puls).

Symptoms in Kent's Repertory	**Page**
Eye, Pupils, insensitive to light	263
Generalities, Apoplexy	1345
Generalities, Catalepsy	1347
Generalities, Collapse	1350
Generalities, Cyanosis/in infants	1356
Generalities, Faintness, excitement/hysterical	1360
Generalities, Narcotics agg.	1375
Generalities, Pulse, imperceptible, almost	1395
Generalities, Reaction, lack of vital	1397
Generalities, Shocks from injury	1399
Generalities, Weakness, rapid	1418
Generalities, Weakness, sudden	1419

SINUSITIS

Sinusitis is caused by a swelling of the mucosal tissue that lines the inside of the nose. This commonly encountered condition is often seen following an upper respiratory illness such as a cold or flu. The swelling of the tissue blocks the opening to the sinuses located in the cheek bones, forehead, and deep within the nose itself, causing increased pressure, pain, swelling and tenderness.

Infection will occur later if the pressure is not relieved and bacteria or viruses have a chance to multiply. Complication of **meningitis** or **facial bone inflammation** rarely occur, but need to be kept in mind if the condition persists and continues to get worse. **Chronic sinusitis** may also be due to an allergic reaction to environmental toxins. Foods such as wheat, dairy, refined sugars and white flours may be at cause. Sensitivity to dust, pollens, animals or dry climate may also contribute.

Using over-the-counter medicines to relieve symptoms will not, in the long run, eliminate the cause. Persistent sinusitis can lead to scarring of the tissue, overgrowth and permanent damage. Treatment becomes more difficult when this has occurred, and surgical repair may be necessary.

Arsenicum alb (3)

Thin, **watery**, **excoriating discharge**; nose feels **stopped up**; sneezes without relief; hayfever and coryza < in open air > indoors; **burning**, bleeding; cold sores in nose; sneezing with coryza but stopped up nose; sensitive smell; **burning thirst**, **craves warm drinks**, **drinks little and often**; **many fears**; **anxiety**; **restlessness**; **chilly**.

< cold, **ice drinks**, **foods**, air	**> hot applications**; **food**
< midnight; after 2 AM	> warm drinks; motion
< vegetables; **drinking**	**> elevating head**
< eruptions; suppressed	> sitting erect; company

< tobacco; **exertion**; seashore
< right side
> sweating

Kali bic (3)

Pressure, fullness and pain at root of nose, sticking pain in nose; pain in small spots; headache > with discharge of fluids; **ulcerated septum**; round ulcer; **fetid smell, discharge is thick, ropy, greenish-yellow**; **tough, elastic plugs** from nose which leave a raw surface; inflammation extends **to frontal sinuses**, with distress and fullness at root of nose; **postnasal drip** (Hydr); **loss of smell**; much hawking due to difficulty with dislodging mucous; cannot breathe through nose; **coryza with nasal obstruction**; **violent sneezing**; profuse, watery nasal discharges; chronic frontal sinus inflammation; little fever but much weakness; **mucus tastes sticky**; **aching and fullness in glabella**; **bones and scalp feel sore**; pains migrate quickly; nasal polyps; thirst; **chilly**.

< cold, damp, air, undressing
< AM, after sleep, 2–3 AM
< protruding tongue; hot weather
< alcohol; beer; suppressed catarrh
> heat, motion

Mercurius (3)

Incessant, from surgery, **nostrils raw, ulcerated**; swelling of nasal bones; discharge is bloody, yellow-green, fetid, pus-like; acrid coryza, thick and does not run; pain and **swelling of nasal bones**; **caries with greenish fetid ulceration**; nosebleed at night; copious discharge of corroding mucus; sneezing **in sunshine**; pains stick to one point; weakness; exhaustion; colds travel upwards; **easy, profuse sweat** without relief; **thirsty**; chilly; frontal sinuses.

< night; sweating, heated
< lying on right side
< extremes of temperature; sensitive to drafts; weather changes, cold damp weather
< wet feet; firelight
< warm room, bed
> moderate temperatures

Natrum carb (2)

Constant coryza; nasal obstruction; **catarrh**, **foul smell of nasal secretion**; many troubles of external nose (Caust); **posterior nasal catarrh**, **hawking**; **much mucus from throat**, **< slightest draft**; headache; **< from sun**; violent sneezing; averse to milk; oversensitive to music, open air, noise; cross; irritable; thirsty.

< heat; sun, weather, light	> motion; rubbing
< 5 AM; music; sitting	> eating; sweating
< mental exertion; milk	> boring in ears and nose
< dietary errors; onanism	
< drafts; thunderstorms	
< weather changes	

Natrum mur (3)

Violent, **fluent coryza**, lasts from 1–3 days then stoppage of nose which makes breathing difficult; thin, watery discharge, **like raw white of egg**; colds that begin with sneezing; **loss of smell and taste**; internal soreness of nose, dryness; frontal sinus inflammation, **thirsty**, chilly.

< 9–11 AM; sun; after menses	> open air; sweating
< alternate days; lying down	> rest; cool bathing
< heat, of sun	> before breakfast, missing a meal
< dampness	> deep breathing
< exertion; eyes; mental	> lying on right side
< violent emotions; sympathy	> tight clothing; pressure against back
< puberty; noise; music	
< warm room; seashore	

Nux vomica (3)

Stuffed-up, **especially at night**; **stuffy colds**, **snuffles** after exposure to dry cold; fluent coryza during the day; **stuffed-up outdoors**; alternates between nostrils; nose bleeds in AM (Bry); acrid discharge but with stuffed-up feeling; frontal headache with desire to press hard against something; nostrils are sore; **angry**; **impatient**; **irritable**; **easily chilled**, **cannot uncover**; **chilly**; thirsty.

< **cold**, **open air**, drafts,
< **uncovering**
< **coffee**, alcohol, drugs
< sedentary habits; overeating
< mental exertion; fatigue; vexation
< **early** AM, disturbed sleep
< slightest noise; odors; touch
< **pressure** of clothes; anger

> **free discharges**
> naps
> wrapping head; rest
> hot drinks; milk
> moist air
> evenings
> strong pressure

Pulsatilla (3)

Coryza; stoppage of right nostril, especially in morning, evening; pressing pain at root of nose; loss of smell (Nat m); large green fetid scales in nose; yellow bland mucus, abundant in AM; soreness of nasal bones; condition better in open air; bad smells, as of old catarrh; **profuse**, **thick**, **bland discharge**; **thirstless**; **short of breath**, **chilly**; **shifting symptoms** which rise to a sudden pitch then cease; anosmia; pale face; pains extend to face and teeth; frontal and supraorbital pains; sad, **weepy**, **wants consolation**, to be held; very sensitive.

< **warmth**, **air**, **room**, **bed**
< **evening**, **suppressions**
< beginning motion
< **rich foods**, **fats**
< **puberty**, **pregnancy**
< getting feet wet
< before menses
< allowing feet to hang down

> **cold**, **fresh air**
> **erect posture**
> uncovering
> gentle motion; weeping
> cold food and drink

Sepia (3)

Thick, **greenish discharge**, thick plugs and crests in nose, **yellowish saddle across nose**; atrophic catarrh with greenish crests from anterior nose, pain at root of nose; chronic catarrh, **especially postnasal**, dropping heavy, lumpy discharges, must be hawked through mouth; sensitive to pain, irritable, averse to family, to sympathy; indifference, poor memory; chilly; string pain from within out; mostly left, with nausea and vomiting.

< cold, **air**, wet, snowy, wind	**> violent motion**
< sexual excesses; washing	> warmth; cold drinks
< before menses; pregnancy	> pressure; cold bath
< AM & PM; after first sleep	> drawing limbs up
< left side; after sweating	> after sleep
< before a thunderstorm	

Silicea (3)

Itching at point of nose; frontal and maxillary, forehead pains; dry, hard crusts form which **bleed when loosened**; nasal bones sensitive; sneezing in AM; nose obstructed with loss of smell; perforated septum; swelling in glabella; discharge is purulent, yellow, green, fetid and may contain blood; are usually bland; vertigo from looking up; **very sensitive**; frothy nasal discharge; **foul foot sweats**; **chilly**, fair complexion; want of grit; **ill effects of vaccination**; **thirsty**; **chilly**.

< cold, air, damp	**> warm, wraps to head**
< uncovering, cold bathing	> profuse urination
< checked sweat; washing	> summer
< new moon; night; alcohol	> wet; humid weather
< mental exertion; in AM	
< lying on left side	

Sensitive to noise, light, jarring spine, excitement

Consider:

Calcarea carb (3)

Nostrils sore, ulcerated, dry; stoppage of nose; fetid yellow discharge; offensive odor in nose; swelling at root of nose; coryza, **takes cold at every change of weather**; catarrhal symptoms with hunger; coryza alternates with colic; **sour discharges**, **head sweats**; **dilated pupils**; **enlarged glands**; chill with thirst; internal heat, externally cold; **thirsty**; **chilly**.

Hydrastis (2)

Thick, tenacious, secretion from posterior nares to throat; watery, **excoriating** discharge; ozena, with ulceration of septum; blows nose all the time; yellow, acrid, ropy secretions; sense of raw burning; shallow ulcers; bloody crusts in nose; < inhaling air; < cold air; > open air.

Natrum ars (3)

Watery discharge drops into throat; **feels stopped**; **pain at root of nose**; dry crusts which leave raw mucous membranes when removed, postnasal drip of thick, bland, yellowish mucus; **crusts in nose**; thirsty, chilly.

Oscillococcinum—suggested for early stages of sinusitis, if due to Influenza.

Sulphur (3)

Stuffy nose indoors; imaginary foul smells; **alae red and scabby**; **chronic dry catarrh**; **dry scabs and easy bleeding**; foul, acrid or blood-streaked discharge; nose obstructed on alternate sides; **thirsty**; chilly.

Symptoms in Kent's Repertory	**Page**
Head, Pain, frontal sinuses, chronic coryza	161
Nose, Catarrah, extends to frontal sinuses/post nasal	325
Nose, Coryza, fever, with/sore throat, with	328
Nose, Discharge, posterior nares, from	333
Nose, Discharge, yellow/green, posterior nares from	333
Nose, Fullness, sense of	338
Nose, Obstruction, sensation of	341
Nose, Pain, bones	343
Nose, Pain, root	344
Nose, Smell, wanting, lost	350
Throat, Mucus, drawn from posterior nares	456

SORE THROAT—PHARYNGITIS

Despite what is commonly held to be true, **sore throats** are not caused by the growth of abnormal bacterial or viral organisms but rather are due to an imbalance of the normal microflora of the mouth, nose and throat. This often accompanies a lowered immune function which is the result of toxemia, becoming chilled, dietary imbalances or treatment with antibiotics, which disrupts the micro-organism balance in the throat.

The type and severity encountered will depend upon which organism has gained the upper hand. **Viral sore throats** are almost always less severe and run a milder course than **bacterial infections**.

Infection with a **beta-hemolytic streptococcal** organism is considered problematic due to the possibility of the development of post-streptococcal nephritis several weeks after the infection. This almost never occurs in well-nourished children and is found more often in the undernourished or immuno-compromised.

Diptherial infection, which is rarely encountered, is characterized by the formation of a membrane across the throat which blocks the airway. This can result in airway obstruction if not treated promptly.

Aconite (3)

Sudden onset, **dry** mucous membranes, hot, burning, inflamed, **constricted**; choking with difficulty swallowing; spikes a 104°F temp; skin is hot and dry; **thirsty**; dry cough, hoarseness; **much anxiety**, **restlessness**; **red throat**, numb; tonsils swollen and dry; **after exposure to cold**, **dry wind**.

< noise, light	> open air, repose
< sleeping in sun	> warm sweat
< lying on affected side; music	
< tobacco smoke; dry cold wind	

< violent emotions; **fright**; **shock**
< pressure, touch

Ailanthus (2)

Throat is **swollen**, inflamed, dark red, purplish; **swollen tonsils** with a full feeling; **enlargement of tonsils**, **swelling of the neck**, **parotid**, **submaxillary** and thyroid gland; ulceration of fauces, **tonsils**; hot, tingling feeling in throat, descends into windpipe and may cause a choking feeling with inspiration; raw, tearing sensation in trachea with coughing; **neck feels tender**, **swollen**; **tongue dry**, **brown**; **pain with swallowing**, extends to ears; dry cough; face may appear dark or red and hot with fevers (Bell), later changing to a dusky hue; skin may appear livid, purplish, with miliary rash; pupils dilated (Bell); headache < at back of neck, **stiffness of neck**; streptococcal infections, influenza; thirst for cold drinks; chilly; restless; **weakness**; dizziness.

< pressure of clothes (Lach)

> lying on right side (bronchial affections)

Apis (2)

Edema, redness, burning; < heat and > cold; **uvula hangs down like a bag**; **throat is fiery red and puffy**, leading to a sensation of suffocation (anaphylaxis); sensation as if a splinter in throat; **constriction**, spasm with swallowing which goes to nose; thirstless; throat shiny; glazed; very sensitive to being touched on neck; stinging pain, ulcers of tonsils; **fiery red margin** around leathery membrane; gums and lips swollen; tongue feels scalded.

< heat; **touch**; pressure
< late afternoon; after 4 PM
< after sleeping; right side
< in closed, heated rooms
< suppressed eruptions

> open air
> uncovering
> cold bathing
> cool air
> motion; slight expectoration

Belladonna (3)

Hot, throbbing, dilated pupils; **throat and tongue are bright red**; strawberry tongue; swollen tongue, tonsils bright red with small white patches; throat is glazed and shiny, **constricted**, **cannot drink**

water; swallowing is painful but have constant desire to do so (Merc sol); burning tongue aggravated by liquids (Canth); **redness is < right side**; sensation of a lump in throat; **spasms** in throat; hypertrophy of mucous membranes; tongue is swollen, painful; thirsty; drinks in sips.

< touch; **jar**; **noise**	> semi-erect
< drafts, after noon (3 PM)	> light covering
< lying down; heat	> bending backward
< checked sweat; **light**	> bed rest
< company; pressure	
< motion	

Guaiacum (2)

Worse right side, not as severe as Belladonna; **tonsils are dry** and hot, feel burned; need to drink or swallow; feels like pepper in throat; puffy face, dilated pupils; may have joint pains in fingers; joints < heat; throat feels on fire; rheumatic sore throat, weak throat muscles; pain stitches toward ear; **acute tonsillitis**; syphilitic sore throat; **unclean odor from body**.

< 6 PM to 4 AM	> external pressure
< motion; **heat**; pressure	> cold (locally)
< cold wet weather	> apples
< touch; exertion	
< rapid growth	

Hepar sulph

Later stages, tonsils that **suppurate**; **fish-bone sensation in throat** to ear; **very sensitive to cold**; to examination; irritable; barking cough; perspiration; hawks up mucus; **very sensitive to all impressions**, thirsty, **chilly**.

< becoming cold	**> damp weather**
< cold, **dry wind**	**> wrapping head**
< cool air; drafts; exertion	
< touch; lying on painful side	
< least uncovering; noise	
< warmth; after eating	

Lac caninum

Pain moves left to right (Lach); **glazed, shiny** throat; much inflammation; cannot swallow but desires to; tonsils coated with white patches; mild sore throat before and after menses (chronic); sensitive to touch, painful swallowing, which extends to ears; **symptoms change from side to side**; **stiffness of neck and tongue**; tickling sensation causes cough.

< **touch**; jar; during menses	> cold, cold drinks
< AM of one day, PM of next	> open air
< cold air or wind or drinks	

Lachesis (2)

Begins on left side to right side; < heat and constriction; **pain is < with slightest pressure**; **throat very sensitive**; difficulty breathing, throat closes off; purplish-blue in color; not as swollen as it feels; sensation of a lump in throat which goes up and down when swallowing; tough mucus; **> swallowing solids**; tongue trembles with protrusion; neck is stiff; chronic constipation; **< swallowing liquids**; throat is dry; **pain aggravated by hot drinks**; **pains travel to ear**; swollen tongue; thirsty.

< retarded discharges	**> appearance of discharges**
< in spring	> warm applications
< after sleep; in AM	**> open air**
< on left side	**> cold drinks**
< warm bath; pressure	> hard pressure; bathing part
< hot drinks; closing eyes	
< heat	
< empty swallowing	

Sensitive to: **slight pressure**; noise

Lycopodium (3)

Dryness of throat with no thirst; stitches with swallowing; swelling and suppuration of tonsils, ulceration of tonsils; **begins on right side**; **deposits spread from right to left**; foul odor of mouth (Merc); chilly.

< eating, to satiety
< cold drinks; awaking
< right side; right to left
< 4–8 PM; heat
< hot air; bed
< warm applications
< pressure of clothes

> hot drinks for throat
> motion; urinating
> after 12 midnight
> warm food and drink
> getting cold; being uncovered
> eructations

Mercurius cor (2)

Red, swollen, painful, intense inflammation; painful to swallow; pain mostly postnasal with sharp pain to ears; burning pain with much swelling; > slight external pressure; swollen glands; salivation.

< evenings; night
< acids; after swallowing
< after urinating; stool
< hot, damp; cool nights

> at rest

Mercurius cyan

Diphtheria remedy; raw hoarseness; dryness; looks raw; touching ulcer causes it to bleed; throat is painful from speaking; **necrotic destruction of soft palate and fauces**; intense redness of fauces; difficult swallowing; ulcerations have a gray membrane; < swallowing, speaking.

Mercurius Iod Flav (2)

Only right side; gags on what's brought up; **tongue has a thick yellow base**; posterior fossa dotted with small ulcers; parotid; cervical glands swollen; **constant inclination to swallow**; much tenacious mucus; easily detached patches on posterior fauces; stiffness of neck.

< odors
< lying on left side

> open air
> cold drinks

Mercurius Iod Rub

Worse left tonsil; dark red fauces; similar to Merc IF.

> cold drinks

Mercurius (2)

Much salivation; sweats; night sweats do not relieve; offensive discharges; scalloped tongue; ulcerations of mouth; thick, dry, heavy coated or moist tongue which trembles when stuck out; throat is dusky red, feels raw, burned, dry; **thirsty**; painful swallowing with desire to swallow (Bell); dark red patches on tonsils; enlarged tender cervical glands; **desires cold drinks**; bluish-red swelling of throat; pain stitches into ear on swallowing; < right side; fluids return through nose; inflammation and suppuration with difficult swallowing, **after pus has formed**; loss of voice; burning in throat , **foul breath**; **great thirst with moist tongue**; chilly.

< night, wet; damp	> moderate temperature
< lying on right side; wet feet	
< perspiring; **heated**	
< warm room and bed	
Sensitive to: **drafts** to head, changes of weather; cold, damp weather; heat and cold	

Phytolacca (3)

Pain at root of tongue which travels to ear with swallowing, **throat dark red-blue**; uvula edematous; swollen glands; sensation of a lump in throat (Bell, Lach); burning pain with dryness; **< drinking, especially hot water** (Lach); yellow coat down center of tongue; flushed face; increased fever, feels chilly; aching, restlessness in different parts of the body; < motion but wants to move; **throat feels rough**, **narrow**, **hot**; **swollen tonsils** especially right; thick, tenacious yellowish mucus which is difficult to dislodge; **quinsy**; **tonsils and fauces swollen**; **mumps**; **follicular pharyngitis**; **red tip of tongue** (Rhus t).

< change of weather	> warmth; dry weather
< electric charges	> rest
< rain; **exposure to damp**	> cold drinks
< cold weather; night	> lying on abdomen
< motion; exposure; right side	
< rising up; swallowing	
< hot drinks; heat	

Consider:

Baryta mur

Hypertrophied tonsils with no inflammation; repeated colds; swollen submandibular glands; feels hot and damp at night; flushed face and dry lips; can see veins in back of throat; moderate fever, low-level infections, > sipping cold water, paresis of pharynx and Eustachian tubes, tubes feel too wide open.

Cantharis (1)

Intense burning; sensation as if they drank boiling water; feels like fire; < back of throat; inflammation with rawness and vesicles; intense thirst but will not drink; constriction of larynx with suffocation; loss of voice; **great difficulty swallowing liquids**; **tenacious mucus**; violent spasms produced by touching larynx.

Dulcamara

Sore throat from **cold wet weather**; much postnasal catarrh; yellow mucus and dark red throat, dry and shiny; dry tongue; hoarse voice especially in AM; gets hives, < heat and scratching.

Kali bic (2)

Fauces red, inflamed, dry, rough; relaxed uvula, **edematous and bladder-like**; pseudomembranous deposits on tonsils, soft palate; burning that extends to stomach; tough, stringy discharges from nose and mouth; tongue is mapped, **red**, **shining**, **smooth and dry**.

Nitric acid

Dry throat; pain travels to ears; hawks mucus constantly; white patches and **sharp pains as from splinters** on swallowing; **bloody saliva**; **ulcers of palate**.

Streptococcinum

Consider if person is a **carrier of beta-hemolytic streptococcus**; has periodic sore throats and or constantly running nose and sinus drainages; if tonsils are hypertrophied and beta strep grows on culture in moderate to large amounts.

Symptoms in Kent's Repertory **Page**

STYES—BLEPHARITIS

Styes are caused by an inflammation of one of the meibomian or sebaceous glands which line the edge of the eyelid. The condition may occur by itself or along with **conjunctivitis** or **iritis**. Caution must be taken when treating a stye, as the release of exudate with homeopathic treatment may cause an infection.

Generally the presence of styes is not considered a severe condition. If the inflammation does not resolve and begins to spread to the surrounding structures, infection of the eye may occur which needs to be evaluated by a physician to prevent the possibility of blindness.

Conium (3)

Stony-hard indurations; **slightest ulceration or abrasion will cause intense photophobia**; **photophobia with excessive lachrymation**; lids heavy, droop, < outer side; fears being alone; eyes feel crossed; smarting pains < open air; large swelling; burning; thirsty; chilly.

< viewing moving objects	
< alcohol	> letting part hang down
< raising arms; exertion; injury	> fasting; in dark; motion
< night; cold; talking; lying with head low	> pressure

Pulsatilla (3)

Upper left lid usually, toward inner canthi; tend to recur but move from spot to spot; **agglutinated eyelid** in AM; yellow, **bland discharge**; **lids inflamed**, **styes**; **thirstless**.

< heat, **rich foods**; **fats**	**> open air**; motion
< warm room; evenings	> cold applications
< lying on left or painless side	> cold food and drink

> erect posture
> weeping

Sepia (3)

Indurations, associated with prominent Sepia presenting symptoms; aggravation of eye problems in AM and PM; tarsal tumors; hardened indurations; drooping eyelids; chilly.

< cold, **air**; wind; wet, snowy	**> violent motion**
< sexual excesses; before menses	> warmth; cold drinks
< AM & PM; after first sleep	> cold bath
< before thunderstorm	> after sleep

Silicea (2)

Induration after eruptions; recurrent and does not tend to localize in any one place; can recur in same spot; feeling of dryness; sand in eye; angles of eyes affected; averse to light, produces sharp pain; eyes tender to touch; **thirsty**; **chilly**; **swelling of lachrymal duct**.

< cold changes; **air**, **drafts**	**> warm**, **wraps**,
< becoming damp	> profuse urination
< bathing; uncovering	
< cold feet	
< noise; jarring of spine; excitement; light	
< change of moon; night	
< mental exertion	
< suppressed foot sweat	

Staphysagria (3)

Left side more often than right; upper lid more often than lower; tend to cause indurations; begins as a central pimple with smaller ones around it then becomes larger; feels as if a hard substance is underneath; heat in eyes; **recurrent styes**; eyes sunken with blue rings; margins of lids itch; angles of eyes effected, especially inner; dryness of eyes; blepharitis; **very sensitive**; chilly; indignant; **chalazion** (Platanus).

< emotions; chagrin; **vexation**	> warmth; rest; breakfast

< quarrels
< sexual excesses; onanism
< touch; cold drinks; night
< anger; loss of fluids; tobacco

Sulphur (3)

Recurrent in the same place; more in upper lid and toward inner canthi; red margins of lids, **burning**, stinging; yellow or whitish discharge, excoriating; lids strongly agglutinated in AM; ulceration of lid margins; **thirsty**, chilly; heat and **burning in eyes** (Ars. Bell).

< bathing, suppressions
< heated, becoming; rest
< speaking; atmosphere changes
< 11 AM; full moon

> open air; motion
> warm applications
> dry heat; sweating

Consider:

Graphites (3)

Blepharitis; dryness of lids; eczema of lids; fissures of lids; **eyelids red and swollen**; intolerance of artificial light.

Lycopodium (3)

Styes on lids near inner canthi; ulceration and redness of lids.

Symptoms in Kent's Repertory	**Page**
Eye, Agglutinated	235
Eye, Excoriation of lids	240
Eye, Granular lids	240
Eye, Inflammation, lids/margins	243
Eye, Inflammation, meibomian glands	244
Eye, Itching, lids/margin	245
Eye, Redness, lids	264
Eye, Redness, edges of	265
Eye, Styes	266
Eye, Swollen, lids/meibomian glands	267
Eye, Tumors on lids/meibomian/nodules	268

URETHRITIS—
Gonococcal & Non Gonococcal

An **inflammation** of the **urethra** is often accompanied by pain and difficulty with urination, frequency of urination and a discharge, which may be especially evident in the mornings. It often produces more severe symptoms in men than in women due to the nature of the individual genital tracts. In females, it often accompanies infections of the vagina.

Most often the infecting agent is bacterial and/or chlamydia, which if left untreated will spread to other areas of the genital urinary tract and may cause sterility. As a rule, if one partner is infected, so is the other even though they do not have symptoms.

Persistent infections, which do not respond to treatment, must be evaluated by a physician in order to prevent further transmission, scarring and sterility.

Agnus castus (3)

Gleety discharge, yellow discharge; no erections, **impotence**, **parts cold**, **relaxed**; **no desire** (Con, Sabal, Sel); scanty emissions without ejaculation; loss of prostatic fluid on straining; testis swollen, cold, hard, painful; spermatorrhea; history of repeated GC: sexual melancholy; **sadness with impression of speedy death**; **gnawing itching** may be present.

< **venery** (excess sexual activity)

Alumina (3)

Gleety discharge, chronic discharges; excessive desire; involuntary emissions with straining at stool; prostatic discharge; **must strain at stool in order to urinate**; **great exhaustion after menses**; **dryness of mucous membranes**; tickling in sexual organs.

< periodically; in afternoon	> open air
< from potatoes; in AM on awaking	> cold bathing

< warm room; sitting
< after menses; speaking
< artificial foods

> in evening; alternate days
> damp weather
> moderate exertion, temperature

Apis—See under prostatitis.

Berberis—See under prostatitis.

Cannabis sativa (3)

Painful urging; urinates in split stream; stitches in urethra; inflamed sensation with soreness to touch; **burning with urination extends into bladder**, urine scalds, spasmodic closure of sphincter; acute stage of GC; urethra very sensitive; walks with legs apart; dragging in testicles; zigzag pain along urethra; sexual over-excitement; urethral carbuncle; stoppage of urethra by mucus and pus; **scanty burning urine passed drop by drop**; gonorrheal ophthalmia.

< urinating; **darkness**
< exertion; talking; walking
< gonorrhea
< lying down; going upstairs

Cantharis(3)

Strong desire; painful erections; pain in glans penis (Pariera, Prunus); priapism in gonorrhea; **intolerable urging** and tenesmus; cutting pains before, during and after urine; **urine scalds and is passed drop by drop**; **constant desire to urinate**; urine jelly-like, shreddy; bloody urine, dysuria, gripping in bladder; painful swelling in genitals; pulls at penis; sexual irritation; pollutions; **thirsty**; **chilly**.

< urinating
< drinking; cold
< bright objects; touch
< sound of water
< being approached
< drinking coffee, water

> warmth; rest
> rubbing

Digitalis (3)

Nightly emissions, with great weakness of genitals after coitus; gonorrhea; balanitis (Merc), with edema of prepuce; dropsical swelling of genitals; enlarged prostate; hydrocele, scrotum enlarged like a bladder; continued urging to urinate, in drops, dark, hot, burning with sharp cutting or throbbing pain at neck of bladder, **as if a straw were being thrust back and forth**; **urethritis**, phimosis; full feeling after urination; constriction and burning as if urethra too small; early AM erections; swollen prostate; swollen glans (Sulph); profuse, thick, yellow-white gonorrhea; chilly, **thirsty**.

< rising up; exertion; heat	> rest; cool air; open air
< lying on left side; motion	> lying flat on back, still
< smell of food; cold drinks	> with empty stomach
< sexual excesses; music	
< sitting erect; after meals	

Medorrhinum (3)

Nocturnal emissions followed by great weakness; **impotence**; gleet; whole urethra feels sore; urethritis; enlarged and painful prostate with frequent urging and painful urination; painful tenesmus with urinating; **nocturnal enuresis**; urine flows very slowly; scalding urine; sensitive, nervous, hurried; feels far off; things seem strange; chilly.

< damp, cold	**> lying on abdomen**
< touch	> bending backward
< daytime, 3–4 AM	> stretching out; fresh air
< after urination	> being fanned; uncovering
< close room; before storms	> hard rubbing; seaside
< thinking of ailment	> dampness; sunset
< daylight to sunset	
< inland; heat	

Mercurius cor (2)

Extremely swollen penis and testis; **gonorrhea**; red urethral orifice, swollen; sore and hot glans penis; thick **greenish and/or bloody discharge**; intense urethral burning; stabbing pain from urethra to bladder; perspires after urinating, which is passed only in drops causing much pain; fine, painful stinging in left testicle; gonorrheal discharges thin at first, then thick; greenish discharge < night.

< cold; hot days, cool nights	> rest
< evening, night; acids	
< after urinating, stool	

Natrum sulph (3)

Condylomata; soft; fleshy excrescences; greenish discharges; gonorrhea; discharge thick, greenish; little pain; **leukorrhea** yellowish-green; **following gonorrhea in female**; **feels every change from dry to wet**; heat with aversion to uncovering.

< damp, weather, night air, cellars	> open air
< lying on left side	> change of position
< injuries; head	> dry weather
< lifting; touch; pressure	> pressure
< late evening; wind; light	
< music	

Petroselinum (3)

Burning, tingling, down perineum throughout whole urethra; **sudden urging to urinate**; frequent, voluptuous tickling in fossa navicularis (urethra); **gonorrhea**; **intense biting**, **itching deep in urethra**; milky discharge.

Phosphoric acid (2)

Emissions at night and at stool; seminal vesiculitis (Oxal ac), deficient sexual power; tender testicles, swollen; loss of erection during coitus (Nux v); prostatorrhea, even with passing of stool; eczema of scrotum; edema of prepuce; swollen glans penis; herpes of prepuce; sycotic excrescences (Thuja); **milky urine**; polyuria; **frequent urination at night**; **sleepy by day**; **apathetic**; **debility**; **chilly**.

< loss of fluids; sexual excesses	> warmth; short sleep
< fatigue; fevers; convalescence	> stooling
< emotions; grief, chagrin, shock	
< unhappy love; homesickness	
< drafts; cold; music; talking	
< exertion; being talked to	

Pulsatilla (3)

Orchitis; pain from abdomen to testicles; thick yellow urethral discharge; late stage of gonorrhea; stricture; urine passed only in drops and interrupted stream (Clematis); **acute prostatitis**; pain and tenesmus with urination, **< lying on back**; increased desire to urinate, **lying on back**; burning spasmodic pain in bladder after urination; involuntary loss of urine at night, while coughing; passing gas; **profuse**; **bland**, **thick**, **yellow-green discharges**; gonorrheal ophthalmia; burning down left spermatic cord; enlarged prostate; bloody emissions; **thirstless**.

< warmth, **air**, **room**, **bed**
< getting feet wet
< suppressions; **evening**
< rest
< beginning motion; **lying**, left side
< rich foods, fats, ices, eggs
< puberty; **pregnancy**
< before menses

> cold; **fresh air**, **open air**
> uncovering; weeping
> erect posture; gentle motion
> cold food, drinks

Selenium (3)

Dribbling of semen during sleep; dribbling of prostatic fluid; irritability after coitus; **loss of sexual power** with lascivious fancies; **increases desire**, **decreases ability**; semen thin odorless; sexual neurasthenia; loss of erection with coitus; **hydrocele**; urine dribbles; chronic gleet; thirstless; craves stimulants; debility; sensation as if a biting drop were forcing its way out.

< debilitating causes, **hot days**
< sexual excesses; loss of sleep
< singing; drafts
< after sleep; tea; lemonade

> after sunset
> inhaling cool air

Sepia (3)

Coldness of organs; offensive perspiration; **gleet**; discharge from urethra only during night; **no pain**; complaints from coition; condylomata surround head of penis; involuntary urination **during first**

sleep; **sensation as if a lump internally**; slow urination; cutting before urination; **yellow discharge**; **white discharge**; **mucoid discharge**; indifferent, averse to sympathy; chilly.

< cold, **air**, wind	**> violent motion**; warmth
< wet, snowy	> cold drinks, bathing
< sexual excesses; before menses	> pressure; drawing limbs up
< pregnancy; abortion	> after full sleep
< AM & PM; after first sleep	
< washing; left side; after sweating	
< before thunderstorm	

Silicea (2)

Burning and soreness of genitals, with eruption on inner surface of thighs; chronic gonorrhea, with thick, fetid discharge; elephantiasis of scrotum; sexual erethism; nocturnal emissions; hydrocele; prostatic fluid discharge with straining at stool; milky, acrid leukorrhea during urination; bloody involuntary urination; **foul foot sweat**; **very sensitive**; **chilly**; **thirsty**.

< cold changes, **air**, **drafts**	**> warm**, **wraps** to head
< uncovering, bathing, check sweat	> becoming warm
< nervous excitement; light; noise	> profuse urination
< jarring spine; alcohol	> wet or humid weather
< change of moon; night	
< mental exertion; AM	
< menses; lying on left side	

Sulphur (3)

Stitching pain in penis; **involuntary emissions**; **genitals cold**, **relaxed**, **impotent**; **mucus and pus in urine**; **burning in urethra** during urination which lasts for a long time afterwards; **urgency**, **urinates large amounts of colorless urine**; awakes early AM to urinate.

< suppressions; **bathing**	> open air; motion
< being heated, **bed**, **exertion**	> warm applications
< atmospheric changes	> sweating; dry heat
< 11 AM; full moon; at rest	> lying on right side

Thuja (3)

Inflammation of prepuce and glans; pain in penis; balanitis (Dig, Merc); **gonorrheal rheumatism**; **gonorrhea**; chronic induration of testicles; pain and burning near neck of bladder, with frequent and urgent desire to urinate; prostatic enlargement; **profuse discharge**; **watery discharge**; **yellowish** gleet; burning, sticking, numbing, drawing or wandering pains, < warmth; urine burns; sensation of trickling after urination; small split stream; urethra swollen, inflamed; wart like excrescences, fig warts, condylomata; fixed ideas; hasty and anxious; thirsty; chilly; severe cutting pains after urination (Sars).

< cold, **damp**; at night
< heat of bed; 3 AM & 3 PM
< increasing moon; menses
< urinating; gonorrhea; syphilis
< vaccination; tea; onions
< after breakfast; fat; coffee

> warm, wind, air
> wrapping head; sneezing
> motion; free secretions
> crossing legs; touch
> left side; drawing limbs up

Consider:

Aurum met (3)

Discharge in syphilitics; pain in the testis and spermatic cord, especially the right, which is < night.

Gleety discharge:

Benzoic acid(3)—See under cystitis.

Kali chl (3)—consider if nephritis or chronic nephritis is present; if much albumin and blood is present.

Kali iod (3)

Natrum mur (3)

Gonorrheal discharge:

Calcarea sulph (3)

Cochlearia (3)—Compare Cinnabaris, Sinapis nigra and Capsicum

Cubeb (2)—Urethritis with mucus, especially in women; thick, yellow discharge; cystitis.

Ferrum phos (3)—Urinary incontinence, with irritation of the bladder neck.

Mercurius (3)—Greenish discharge, tinged with blood; nocturnal emissions tinged with blood.

Nitric acid (3)—Soreness and burning in prepuce and glans; sticking pains; see prostatitis.

Senecio (1)—Dull, heavy pains in spermatic cord which extend to the testicles; bloody urination **with much heat**, **urging and pain**; **prostatic enlargement**.

Terebinthina (3)—See cystitis.

Symptoms in Kent's Repertory	**Page**
Bladder, Fullness, sensation of	645
Bladder, Inflammation/neck	646
Bladder, Urging, constant	653
Bladder, Urging, painful	654
Bladder, Urination, interrupted	658
Bladder, Retarded, must wait for urine	660
Bladder,Urination, must press a long time	661
Urethra, Agglutination of meatus	669
Urethra, Discharge, bloody/gleety	669
Urethra, Discharge, gonorrheal	667
Urethra, Discharge, greenish/purulent	671
Urethra, Inflammation	672
Urethra, Itching, gonorrheal/fossa navicularis	672

See **Prostatitis**

WOUNDS

There are several different classifications of **wounds**, each of which carries its own needs for treatment and problems of management. **Abrasions** involve the upper layers of skin only, while an **avulsion** is characterized by the tearing of the skin. A **laceration** is caused by a sharp object which leaves an uneven cut, while an **incision** is caused by an object such as a knife. A **puncture wound** may be caused by any object which pierces the skin and either continues on through or comes out the way it entered.

In all cases, **infection is a concern**, as the protective covering of the skin to environmental bacteria has been removed. With deeper cuts and lacerations, damage to underlying structures such as nerves, tendons, veins and arteries may have occurred. Bleeding either into the underlying tissues or out the wound may be present. A spurting of blood denotes an **arterial laceration** and is considered a medical emergency. A steady, oozing type of flow is from a **vein** and is more easily managed with pressure.

Any laceration or wound needs to be evaluated by medical personnel in addition to treatment with homeopathic medicines.

Arnica (2)

Wounds, **contusions**, **bruises**, which bleed freely; cuts; splinters, bullet wounds; **tendency to bleed and bruise**, may be accompanied by a high fever or a chronically low fever; **bruised and sore feeling following trauma**; grief and/or shock from trauma; see shock.

< motion; touch

Calendula

Lacerated and **suppurating**, **raw**, **open** and **inflamed wounds**; **abscesses**, **boils**, **burns**, **carbuncles**, **fistula**, **whitlow**; when fever is present (Arn), **patient is very sensitive to open air**; helps abscess formation, especially if a warm solution is used; hemostatic in tooth extractions; calendula tincture is reported to work better if warmed rather than cold; **best used in the tincture**, **succus form or 3x potency**.

Hypericum

Crush injuries, **lacerations of fingers**, **tips**; **painful**, penetrating wounds; may have spasms from the injury; splinters, bullet wounds, **puncture wounds** (Led), ***wounds which are excessively painful; crush injuries of the tail bone***, which are **painful**; injuries from forceps deliveries; **lancinating pains along nerves**, tingling, burning pains of nerves, numbness; **crawling sensations in hands or feet**; prostration from blood loss (Phos); wounds which are very tender and < touch.

< touch; **jarring**
< cold

Lachesis (2)

Wounds which are **slow to heal** (Nit ac), **dissecting** wounds (Anth, Apis, Arn, Led, Pyrogen); bites of poisonous animals (Led); **bluish hue** around wound or ulcer; inflammation of lymphatics leading from the wound; see abscesses.

Ledum (3)

Wounds which become cold; **bites of poisonous animals** (Lach), puncture wounds, **ill effects from puncture wounds**; cuts; painful splinters, **penetration wounds**, especially of the palms and soles; stinging pains, pains tend to travel upward; swelling; ***part feels cold but patient does not want it covered***, **is > cold applications**, < warmth; follows Arnica well for bruises which are slow to heal.

< warmth — **> cold**
< night

Nitric acid (1)

Wounds which are slow to heal (Lach), **penetrating**; painful wounds, from splinters, with shooting, stinging, **sticking pains**, **splinter-like pains**; pains appear and disappear quickly; **suppuration**;

may have a sensation of a band around the part; wounds that sting, burn and bleed easily, especially after being touched; wound is very sensitive.

Phosphorus (2)

Wounds which bleed freely, will heal then break open again; bleeding, effects of chronic loss of blood from the wound; bloody discharges; **petechiasis**; **bruising**; numbness of extremities; bone inflammation and necrosis, osteomyelitis; shooting pains; symptoms may come on suddenly; see hemorrhages. (Consider Phosphoric acid in young persons whose wounds, abscesses, boils, etc., fail to heal while they are in a growth phase.)

Staphysagria (2)

Pains from lacerations, **surgical incisions**, **especially following abdominal operations**, from stretching of sphincters; **painful** splinters, stab wounds; stinging pains; post-operative wounds which are slow to heal; good for incarcerated flatus post-operatively (Raphanus); lacerations of the cornea (Arn, Led, Symphytum); tooth pain following extraction; patient is often **hypersensitive to pain**, to what others say about her. (Consider the use of Arnica, Phosphorus & Rhus tox pre-operatively, Arnica, Bellis per for GYN surgery, and Phosphorus post-operatively. Also consider Chloroform if this was used for anesthesia.)

< touch	> warmth

Strontia carb

Similar to Carbo veg but is < cool air and > warmth; hemorrhages, oozing of dark blood from mucous membranes following injuries or surgery, especially of the nose; depletion following or from hemorrhages (China); bright colors which change, dance before eyes, green spots, photophobia following surgery; **shock following surgery**; debilitated, usually < on right side; good high blood pressure medicine, flushing of the face with pulsation of vessels; very sensitive to cold.

< cold	**> warmth**
< bleeding	
< beginning to move	

Sulphuric acid (2)

Wounds which fail to heal; **prolonged ecchymosis**; **prostration** from injuries, wounds; gangrene following mechanical injuries; intraocular bleeding following a blow to the eye (Lach, Merc c, Phos for retinal bleeding, bleeding from the eye); scars are red and blue and very painful; follows Arnica well for bruises (Ledum); patient may be irritable, hurried.

< mechanical injuries
< excess heat
< touch, pressure

> warmth; rest

FOREIGN BODIES

Hepar sulph

Felons, **suppurations**, especially from foreign bodies; **felons which occur every spring**; patient is **very sensitive to touch and cold**; see abscesses.

Silicea

Felons, splinters, stab wounds; stinging pains; **good for expulsion of foreign bodies**, give low and frequently; acts to ripen abscesses (see abscesses); **violent sticking pains** (Nit ac); resorption of fibrous tissue, scar tissue; bone fragments which have not healed or been resorbed; patient is chilly, **very sensitive to the cold** (Hepar) and can be prostrated which may become > with expulsion of the object; see abscesses.

FRACTURES

Calcarea phos (3)

Non-union of fractures (Symph), bone disease; open fontanelles; poor bone development, softness of bones; joint and bone pains; **soft**, **thin** and **brittle bones**; hip joint disease, spina bifida, tuberculosis of the spine; exostosis; **swollen glands**; chilly; (consider Calc carb).

< weather changes
< dentition

Hekla lava

For fractures which heal with nodosities, excessive callosity or exostosis; especially of the jaw; bone tumors, osteosarcoma; inflammations, osteitis, periostitis, abscesses of gums, **enlargement of maxillary bone**; necrosis, especially following mastoid operations; for alternate use with Manganum in osteoarthritis.

Ruta (1)

Good for **damage to the periosteum** (Symph) or **tendons**; pain feels as if it is deeper in the bone, joint; **soreness of tendons**; stiffness of joints which are < lying still and > with movement (Rhus t); bones are < touch; **pains in thigh from stretching**; patient may be restless; follows Arnica well for sprains.

Symphytum (2)

Contusions (Arnica); wounds which penetrate to and involve the bone; **cartilage or bone injuries**, **periosteal injuries** (Ruta); **fractures which fail to heal** (Calc p); sticking, pricking pains, which remain after the wound has healed; **poor callus formation** on X-ray; soreness of bones which is < touch; psoas abscesses; **eye pain following a blow**, see eye injuries. (Several authors considered this to be the number-one remedy for fractures and often gave it in both homeopathic and material doses. My own experience verifies their findings.)

Symptoms in Kent's Repertory	**Page**
Skin, Ecchymosis	1308
Skin, Erysipelas, gangrenous	1323
Skin, Gangrene, from burns or sores	1325
Skin, Swelling, bluish-black	1332
Generalities, Cyanosis	1356
Generalities, Dropsy, external	1356
Generalities, Hemorrhage, blood does not coagulate	1365
Generalities, Indurations	1367

REFERENCES

PROPHYLACTICS IN HOMEOPATHY, Dr. Y. R. Agrawal, Vijay Publications, New Delhi, 1987

CHARACTERISTICS OF THE HOMEOPATHIC MATERIA MEDICA, 2nd Edition, H. Barthel M.D., Barthel & Barthel Publishers, Germany, 1987

MATERIA MEDICA WITH REPERTORY, O.E. Boericke M.D., Boericke & Runyon, Philadelphia, PA, 1927

SYNOPTIC KEY, C.M. Boger M.D., J.Jain Pub. Co., New Delhi, India, 1931

EMERGENCY HOMEOPATHIC FIRST AID: A Quick Reference Handbook, P. Chavanon M.D. & R. , Levannier M.D., Thorsons Publishers Ltd., England, 1977

A STUDY on MATERIA MEDICA and REPERTORY, N.M. Choudhuri M.D., B. Jain Publishers, New Delhi, 1929

COUGH and EXPECTORATION, A REPETORIAL INDEX of THEIR SYMPTOMS, George H Clark M.D., 1st Indian Edition, Roy Publishing House, Calcutta, 1962

DECACHORDS—A CONCISE GUIDE TO THE HOMEOPATHIC MATERIA MEDICA, A.G. Clarke, London, 1913

DICTIONARY OF THE MATERIA MEDICA 3 vol., J.H. Clarke M.D., Health Science Press, Devon, England, 1977

AN OBSTETRIC MENTOR: A Handbook of Homeopathic Treatment Required During Pregnancy, **Parturition and the Puerperal Season**, Clarence M. Conant M.D., Economic Homeo Pharmacy, Calcutta, 1884

EVERYBODY'S GUIDE to HOMEOPATHIC MEDICINE, Stephen Cummings M.D., Dana Ullman M.P.H., North Atlantic Books, Berkeley, 1989

SELECT YOUR REMEDY, Rai Bahadur Das, 4th Edition, Vishwamber Homeopathic Dispensary, New Delhi, India, 1981

THE AMERICAN ILLUSTRATED MEDICAL DICTIONARY, W. A. Dorland, A.M., M.D., F.A.C.S., 21st Edition, W.B. Saunders & Company, 1949

TUTORIALS on HOMEOPATHY, Dr. Donald Foubister BSc., MB., ChB., DCH., FFHom, Beaconsfield Publishers Ltd., England, 1989

STAUFFERS HOMOOPATHISCHES Tashchenblach Uberaibitring:, Dr. med K.H. Gebharrdt, Haug Verlag, Heidelberg, 1984

FIRST AID HOMEOPATHY in accidents and ailments, D.M. Gibson M.B., B.S., F.R.C.S., F.F. Hom., 10th Edition, The British Homeopathic Association, London, 1983

THE APPLICATION OF THE PRINCIPLES AND PRACTICE OF HOMEOPATHY TO OBSTETRICS, H. Guernsey M.D., 3rd Edition, Hahnemann Publishing House, 1883

KENT'S MINOR WRITINGS on HOMEOPATHY, K.H. Gypser M.D. (Ed), Haug Publishers, Heidelberg, 1987

PREHOSPITAL EMERGENCY CARE & CRISIS INTERVENTION, 2nd Edition, B. Hafen & K. Karren, Morton Publishing Co., Colorado, 1983

THE HOMEOPATHIC TREATMENT of CHILDREN—Pediatric Constitutional Types, Paul Herscu N.D., North Atlantic Books, Berkeley, 1991

PROCEEDINGS of the 1989 PROFESSIONAL CASE CONFERENCE, International Foundation for Homeopathy, Seattle, Wash.

PROCEEDINGS of the 1990 PROFESSIONAL CASE CONFERENCE, International Foundation for,Homeopathy, Seattle, Wash.

PROCEEDINGS of the 1991 PROFESSIONAL CASE CONFERENCE, International Foundation for,Homeopathy, Seattle, Wash.

HOMEOPATHY IN PAEDIATRIC PRACTICE, Hedwig Imhauser M.D., Haug Publishers, Germany, 1988

MATERIA MEDICA OF THE NEW HOMEOPATHIC REMEDIES, Dr. O. A. Julian, Beaconsfield, Publishers LTD., U. K., 1984

LECTURES ON HOMEOPATHIC MATERIA MEDICA, J.T. Kent M.D., Homeopathic Publications, New Delhi, 1900

REPERTORY OF THE MATERIA MEDICA, 6th Edition, J.T. Kent, A.M., M.D., B. Jain Publishers Pvt. Ltd, New Delhi, 1986,

KENT'S REPERTORIUM GENERALE, Kunzli M.D., Barthel & Barthel Publishers, Heilelberg, 1987

HOMEOPATHIC THERAPEUTICS, S. Lillienthal M.D., Boericke & Tafel, Philadelphia, 1878

PRACTICE OF MEDICINE, Walter S. Mills M.D., Boericke & Tafel, Philadelphia, 1915

HOMEOPATHIC THERAPEUTICS IN OPHTHALMOLOGY, John Moffad M.D., B. Jain Publishers, New Delhi, 1916

HOMEOPATHIC MEDICINES FOR PREGNANCY AND CHILDBIRTH, Richard Moskowitz M.D., North Atlantic Books, Berkeley, 1992

FUNDAMENTALS of MATERIA MEDICA, Robin Murphy N.D., Self Publication, 1988

LEADERS IN HOMEOPATHIC THERAPEUTICS, 6th Edition, E.B. Nash M.D, Boericke & Tafel, Philadelphia, 1913

A MANUAL OF HOMEO-THERAPEUTICS, E.A. Neatby M.D., & T.G. Stonham M.D., Foxlee-Vaughan Publishers, London, 1948

MATERIA MEDICA of HOMEOPATHIC MEDICINES, Dr. S.R. Phatak M.D. BS., Indian Books & Periodicals, New Delhi, 1977

RUDDOCK'S FAMILY GUIDE TO HOMEOPATHY AND HEALTH, E. H. Ruddock M.D., Halsey Brothers Co., Chicago, 1902

SIMILLIMUM—JOURNAL OF THE HANP, Winter 1991, Vol IV #1

SIMILLIMUM—JOURNAL OF THE HANP, Summer 1991, Vol IV #2

ELEMENTS OF HEALING AND THE SEVEN PLANETARY METALS, R. Stewart, N.D, Unpublished, 1987

BETTER HEALTH THROUGH NATURAL HEALING, Dr. Ross Trattler, Mc Graw-Hill Co., 1985

A DICTIONARY OF HOMEOPATHIC MEDICAL TERMINOLOGY, Jay Yasgur R.Ph., MSc., Van Hoy Publishers, Greenville, PA, 1990

WEBSTER'S NEW WORLD DICTIONARY of the American Language, Second College Edition, Simon & Schuster, 1980

LECTURE & SEMINAR NOTES FROM THE FOLLOWING:

Steven Albin, N.D.
Prem Dev GHMS, N.D.
Durr Elmore D.C., N.D.
Francisco Eizayaga, M.D.
Paul Herscu, N.D.
Martin Milner, N.D.
Roger Morrison, M.D.
Richard Moskowitz, M.D.
Robin Murphy, N.D.
Ravinder Sahni, D.C., N.D.
Andre Saine, N.D.
Mr. George Vithoulkas

GLOSSARY

Adynamic Fevers: a fever with nervous depression, feeble pulse, and a clammy skin; also termed asthenic fever.

Agglutinated: stuck together, as with glue or substance which causes stickiness.

Aggravated: to make worse, more burdensome.

Air Hunger: a lack of oxygen to the tissues,resulting in a blueness of the extremities, lips and mucous membranes; often accompanied by extreme efforts on the part of the person to be able to breathe.

Alae Nasi: the flap on the outside of each nostril.

Ameliorated: to make better, to improve.

Anteversion: the forward tipping or tilting of an organ; usually pertaining to a uterus which is tipped forward.

APGAR Score: score assigned to newborn infants at one and five minutes of life to assess their ability to survive outside the womb.

Appendicitis: an inflammation of the vermiform appendix.

Astringent: causing contraction and arresting discharges; usually a topical agent.

Besotted Look: a silly or foolish look.

Blepharitis: inflammation of the eyelids.

Bronchitis: an inflammation of the bronchial tree.

Cachectic: as pertains to cachexia; see cachexia.

Cachexia: a profound and marked state of general ill health and malnutrition; may accompany a variety if diseases or conditions.

Canthi: pertaining to the canthus; see canthus.

Canthus: the angle at either end of the slit between the eyelids; either the outer or inner.

Carphologia: the involuntary picking at the bed clothes seen in fevers and in conditions of great exhaustion.

Catarrh: inflammation of a mucus membrane with a free discharge, especially of the air passages of the head, throat and respiratory passages.

Chalazion: a small tumor of the eyelid, formed by blockage of secretions of the meibomian gland.

Chemosis: excessive edema of the ocular conjunctiva, whether inflammatory or not.

Chorea: a convulsive and nervous disease characterized by involuntary and irregular jerking movements.

Choreic: as pertaining to chorea; see chorea.

Clonic: as pertaining to clonus; see clonus.

Clonus: spasm in which rigidity and relaxation succeed each other.

Colic: pain in a tubular organ such as the intestines, colon, bile ducts or ureters; used primarily in reference to abdominal pains, especially those in infants and children.

Colitis: inflammation of the colon.

Conjunctivitis: inflammation of the delicate membrane which lines the eyelids and covers the eyeball.

Criencephalique: a piercing cry due to irritation of the covering of the brain.

Croup: a disease characterized by laborious and suffocative breathing, laryngeal spasm and sometimes with local membranous deposits.

Cystocele: a herniated protrusion of the urinary bladder.

Dentition: the cutting of teeth.

Dropsical: pertaining to dropsy, the abnormal accumulation of serous fluid in the tissues or body cavity, resulting in a swollen and bloated appearance.

Dysentery: abdominal pain accompanied by frequent stools with blood and mucus.

Dysmenorrhea: painful and difficult menstruation.

Dyspepsia: impairment of the stomach to digest food, often accompanied by excessive acidity.

Dysphagia: difficulty in swallowing.

Dyspnea: difficult or labored breathing.

Edema: an abnormal accumulation of fluid in the cells and tissues.

Enuresis: the loss of urine due to inability to control its flow.

Epigastrium: the upper middle portion of the abdomen, over or in front of the stomach.

Epileptiform: resembling epilepsy or its manifestations; recurring in severe and sudden paroxysms.

Epistaxis: bleeding from the nose.

Eructations: to belch, burp.

Eustachian tube: the tube that runs from the middle ear to the throat which allows for an equalling of pressure.

Excoriating: to strip, scratch, abrade, chafe or rub off the skin.

Exudates: the outpouring of an adventitious substance such as pus or sebum, from the tissues.

Fetid: to stink; having a bad smell.

Fig Warts: verruca acuminata; a moist, pointed, cauliflower-like venereal wart.

Gastralgia: pain in the stomach.

Gastritis: inflammation of the stomach lining.

Generals: pertaining to symptoms existing or occurring extensively; common; widespread.

Glans: the end or head of the penis.

Gleety Discharge: a chronic form of urethral gonorrheal discharge.

Glossitis: inflammation of the tongue.

Gripping Pain: pain as if held tightly by a hand or instrument.

Gyratory Motion: a circular or spiral motion.

High Colored Urine: urine which is a darker yellow colored, usually associated with being highly concentrated.

Hydrocele: a circumscribed collection of fluid, especially in the tunica vaginalis of the testicle or along the spermatic cord.

Impotence: lack of sexual power; usually associated with inability to obtain or maintain an erection.

Inertia Uteri: pertaining to a uterus which has a decreased ability to contract during labor and delivery.

Intraocular: pertaining to the inside chamber of the globe of the eye.

Jaundice: deposition of bile pigment into the skin and sclera of the eye resulting in a yellow discoloration, is associated with liver disease and hyperbilirubinemia.

Lachrymation: the secretion and discharge of tears.

Lancinating: tearing, darting or cutting sharply; used to describe pain.

Laryngitis: an inflammation of the larynx resulting in a decreased ability to speak or use the voice; may have many causes.

Lienteric: diarrhea in which the stools contain undigested food, especially fats.

Loquacious: fond of talking; excessive talkativeness.

Lumbago: rheumatic pain in the lumbar region of the back.

Melancholic: refers to melancholy, a form of insanity marked by a depressed and painful emotional state with abnormal inhibition of mental and physical bodily activity.

Membranous Dysmenorrhea: painful and difficult menstruation that is characterized by membrane like exfoliation from the uterus.

Modalities: a special attribute, emphasis etc. that marks certain individuals, things or groups.

Mucopurulent: containing both mucus and pus.

Necrotic: pertaining to necrosis or the death and dissolution of tissue.

Nervous Erethism: excessive irritability or sensibility of the nervous system; an unusually quick response to stimulus.

Neuralgia: pain in the nerve or nerves or radiating along the course of a nerve.

Nocturnal Enuresis: urinary loss during sleep.

Occipital: pertaining to the occiput or back portion of the skull.

Onanism: withdrawal from sexual intercourse before ejaculation; also means to masturbate.

Opisthotonos: a condition in which the back muscles, the head and lower limbs are bent backward and the trunk arched forward, while the body rests on the head and heels, due to tetanic muscular spasm.

Ophthalmia: severe inflammation of the eye or conjunctiva.

Otorrhea: a discharge from the ear, especially a purulent one.

Ozaena: imperfect recovery from measles or incomplete treatment resulting in a persistent foul ordered nasal discharge; associated with chronic rhinitis and malignant ulcerations of the nasal mucosa.

Pancreatitis: inflammation of the pancreas.

Particulars: pertains to symptoms which are specific; out of the ordinary; unusual; noteworthy.

Parturition: the act or process of giving birth.

Peevish: hard to please; irritable; fretful; cross.

Perineum: the region which lies between the thighs and the anus and penis or vaginal opening.

Pharyngitis: an inflammation of the pharynx; commonly known as a sore throat.

Photophobia: an abnormal intolerance to light. either natural or artificial.

Polyuria: excessive urination.

Priapism: persistent, abnormal erection of the penis.

Prolapse: the falling down or sinking of a part of viscus.

Prostatitis: inflammation of the prostate gland.

Prostration: utter physical or mental exhaustion or helplessness.

Puerperal: women in labor, childbirth.

Purpura Hemorrhagica: the formation of purple patches on the skin and mucous membranes due to subcutaneous extravasation of blood.

Remedy: any medicine or treatment that cures, heals or relieves a disease or bodily disorder or tends to restore health.

Retching: to undergo the straining action of vomiting, without bringing up any matter.

Retroversion: the tipping of an entire organ backwards; usually pertaining to a uterus which is tilted backward in relation to the pelvic axis.

Rheumatoid Diathesis: an inherited condition which makes the person more susceptible to rheumatoid arthritis.

Rubric: a chapter heading, initial letter or specific sentence; denotes sub sections in the repertory which correspond to patient symptoms.

Sacro-iliac Symphysis: the joint or articulation between the iliac and sacral bones and their ligaments.

Sciatica: painful inflammation of the sciatic nerve causing tenderness, paraesthesia of the thigh and leg.

Scrofulous: associated with tuberculosis of the lymph glands and occasionally of the bones and joints resulting in suppuration abscesses and fistulous passages. Persons referred to as scrofulous have a tendency toward such afflictions.

Sensorial: of the senses or sensation; connected with the reception and transmission of sense impulses.

Sinusitis: inflammation of a sinus; usually taken to mean the maxillary, frontal and ethmoid sinuses of the face.

Sordes: foul, brown crusts.

Strabismus: deviation of the eye which the patient cannot over come; sometimes termed "lazy eye" or squint.

Strangulated: to constrict so as to cut off the flow.

Strangury: slow and painful discharge of the urine due to spasm of the urethra and bladder.

Suffocation: the stoppage of respiration; asphyxia; inability to obtain oxygen.

Suppuration: the formation of pus; the act of discharging pus.

Tenesmus: straining, especially ineffectual and painful, at stool or with urination.

Tonic: characterized by continuous tension; as pertains to continuous contraction of the muscles due to nervous system stimulation.

Tumultuous: greatly agitated; wild and uproarious; great emotional disturbance or agitation of the mind or feeling.

Tympanic: like a drum or drum head.

Uremia: the presence of toxic materials in the blood normally excreted by the kidneys, resulting in nausea, vomiting, vertigo, headache, dimness of vision and eventual coma and death.

Urethritis: inflammation of the urinary urethra.

Uvula: a small, fleshy mass hanging from the soft palate above the root of the tongue.

Varicose: an enlarged and tortuous vein or artery.

Vertigo: a sensation as if the external world were revolving around the patient (objective) or as if he himself were revolving in space (subjective).

Vexed: to distress; annoy; afflict; plague; irritate.

Voluptuous: characterized by sensual delights and pleasure, as in voluptuous itching, itching which feels good.

Waterbrash: heartburn; a burning sensation in the esophagus and stomach, with sour eructations; similar to pyrosis.

APPENDIX

ACUTE GASTROENTERITIS FLOW CHARTS

Use the most characteristic situation to direct you to the correct chart.

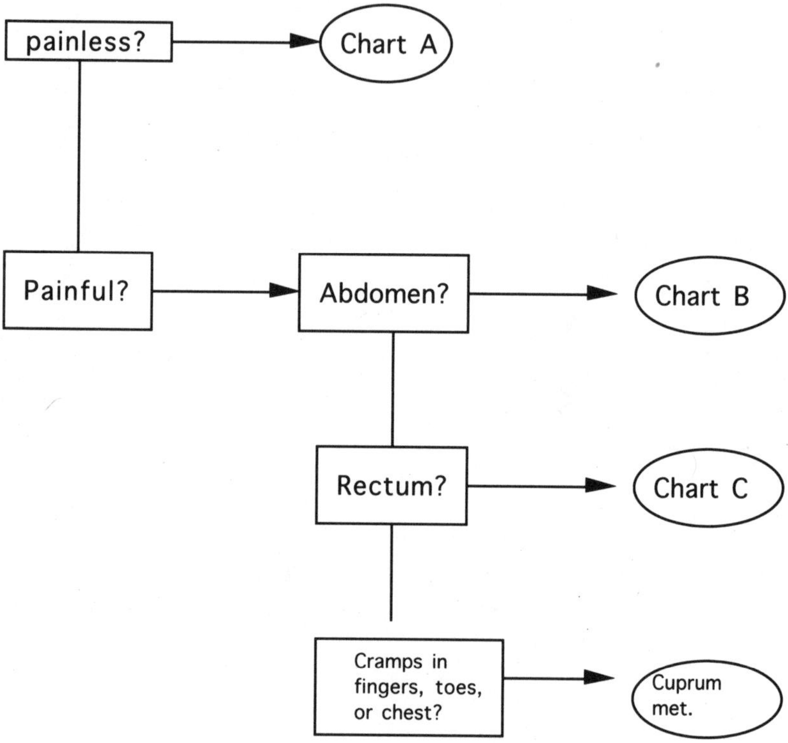

Please note: This information is to be used only under your doctor's supervision.

CHART "A"
PAINLESS DIARRHEA

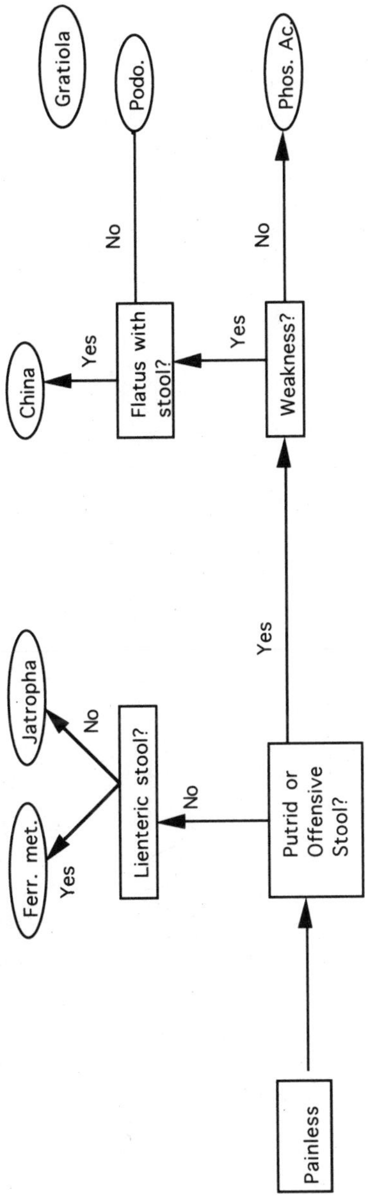

CHART "B"
ABDOMINAL PAIN

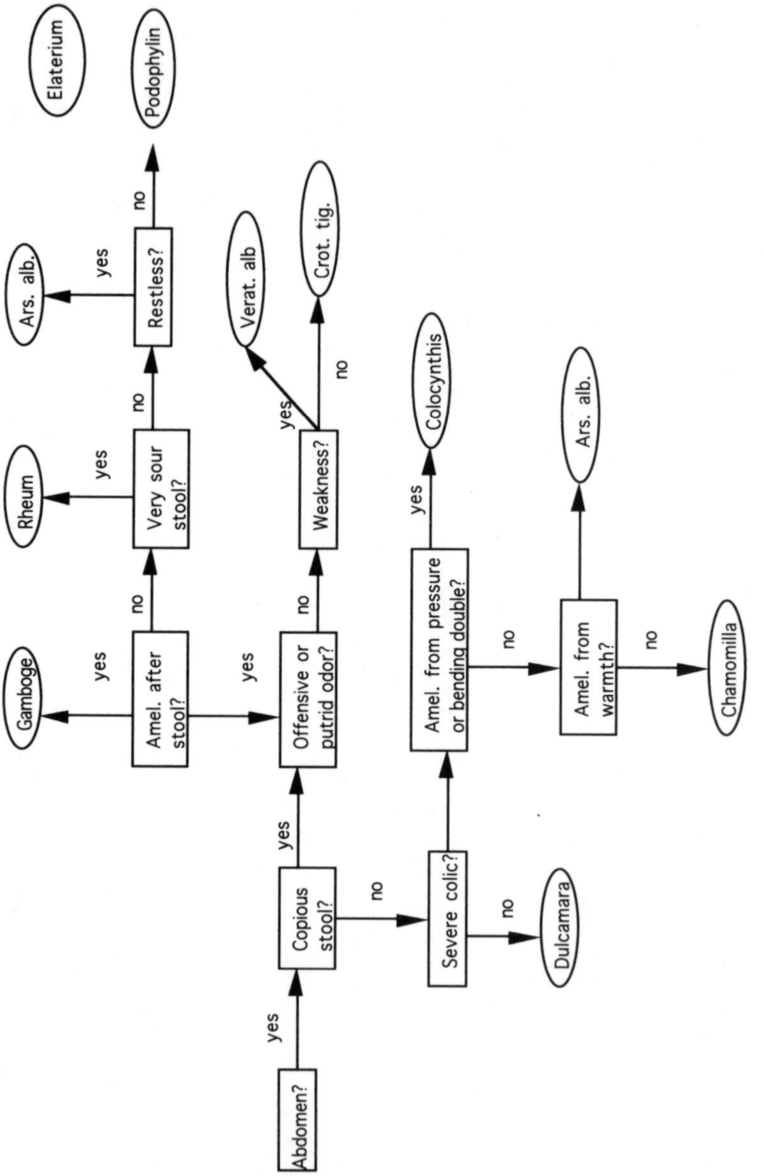

CHART "C"
RECTAL PAIN

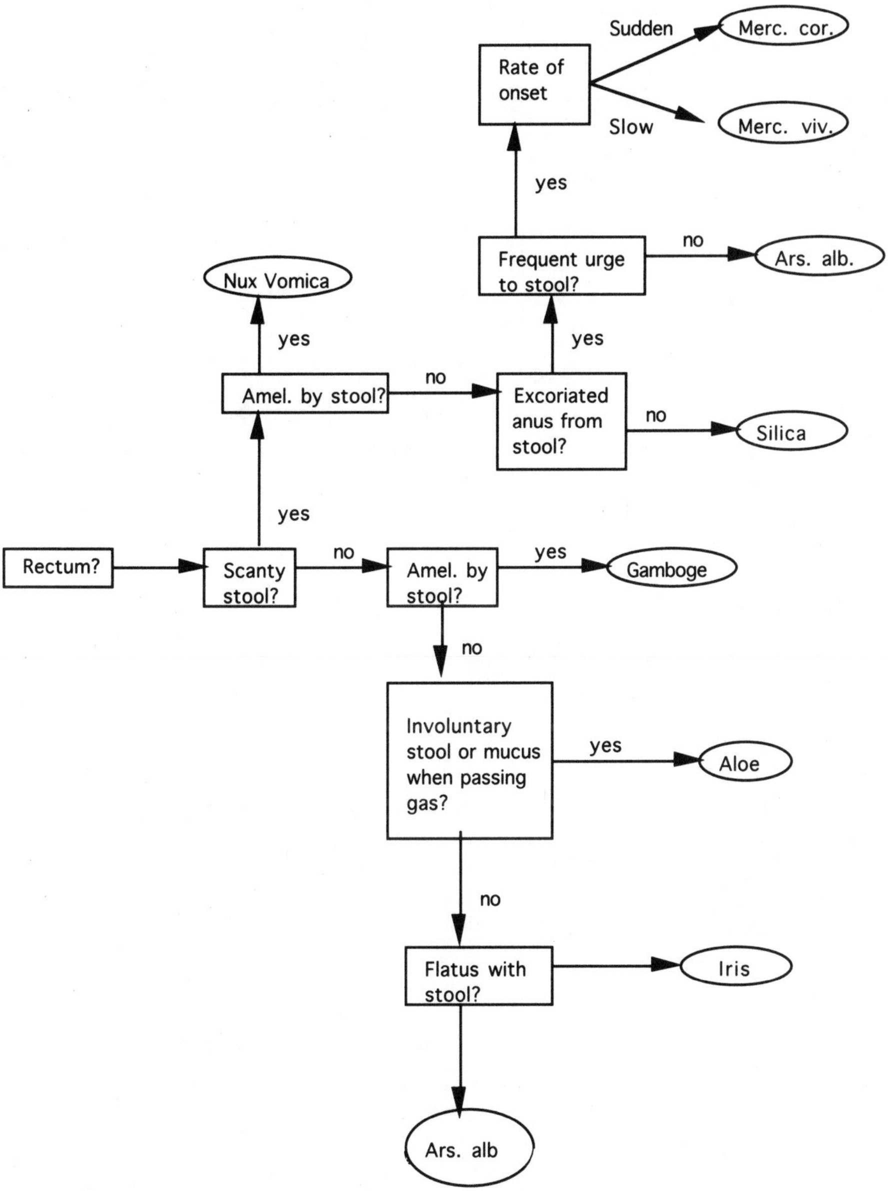

ACUTE CYSTITIS

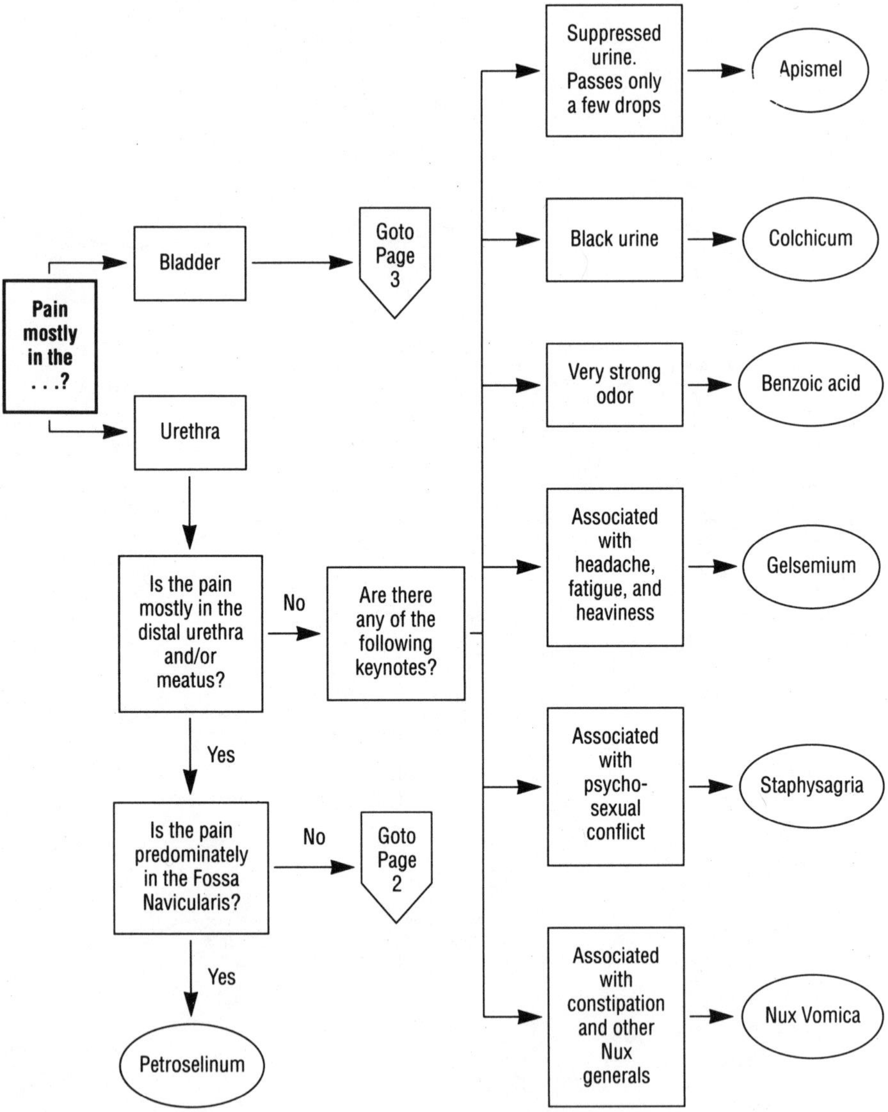

Page 1

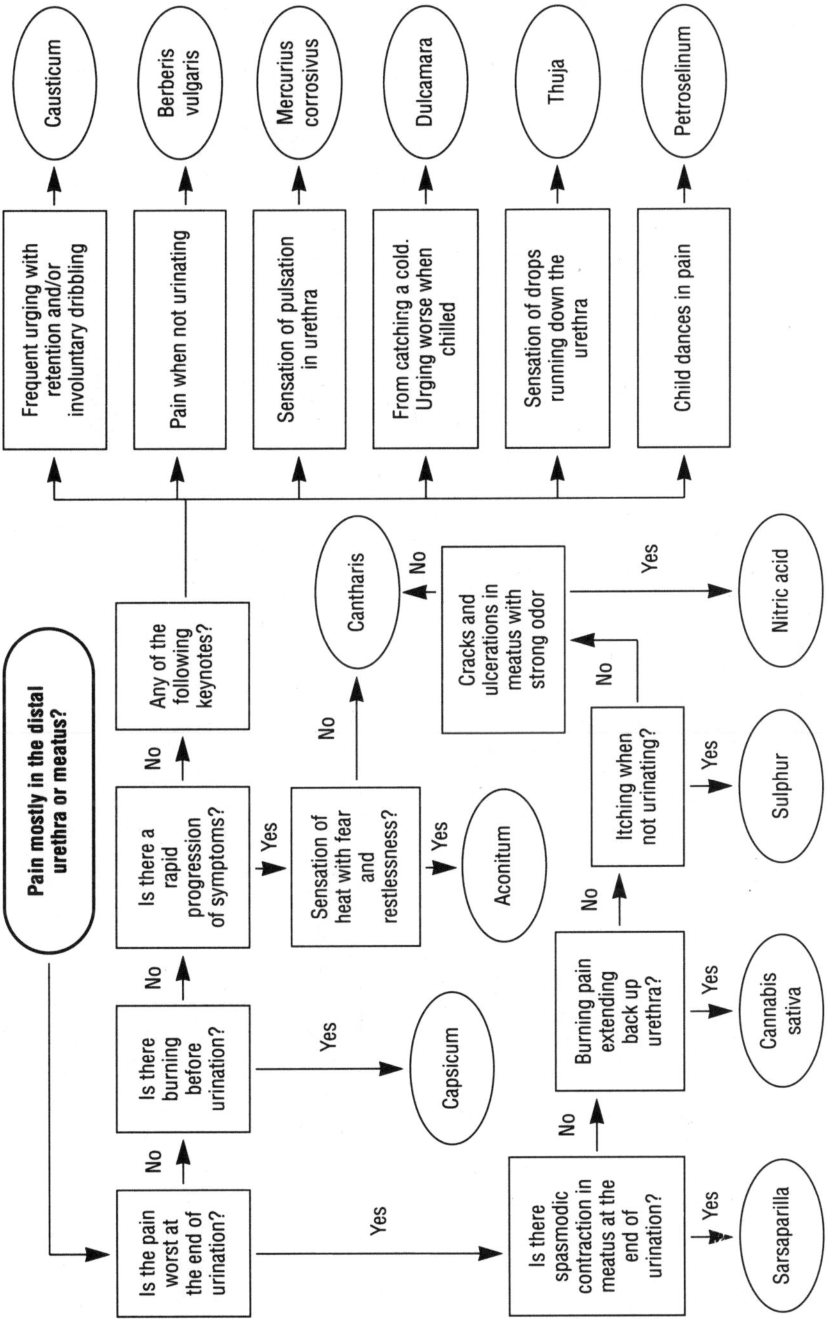
Pain mostly in the distal urethra or meatus?
Is the pain worst at the end of urination?
No
Yes
Is there burning before urination?
Yes
Capsicum
No
Is there a rapid progression of symptoms?
Yes
Sensation of heat with fear and restlessness?
Yes
Aconitum
No
Cantharis
No
Any of the following keynotes?
Frequent urging with retention and/or involuntary dribbling
Causticum
Pain when not urinating
Berberis vulgaris
Sensation of pulsation in urethra
Mercurius corrosivus
From catching a cold. Urging worse when chilled
Dulcamara
Sensation of drops running down the urethra
Thuja
Child dances in pain
Petroselinum
Is there spasmodic contraction in meatus at the end of urination?
Yes
Sarsaparilla
No
Burning pain extending back up urethra?
Yes
Cannabis sativa
No
Itching when not urinating?
Yes
Sulphur
No
Cracks and ulcerations in meatus with strong odor
No
Yes
Nitric acid

Page 2

CYSTITIS FLOW CHARTS

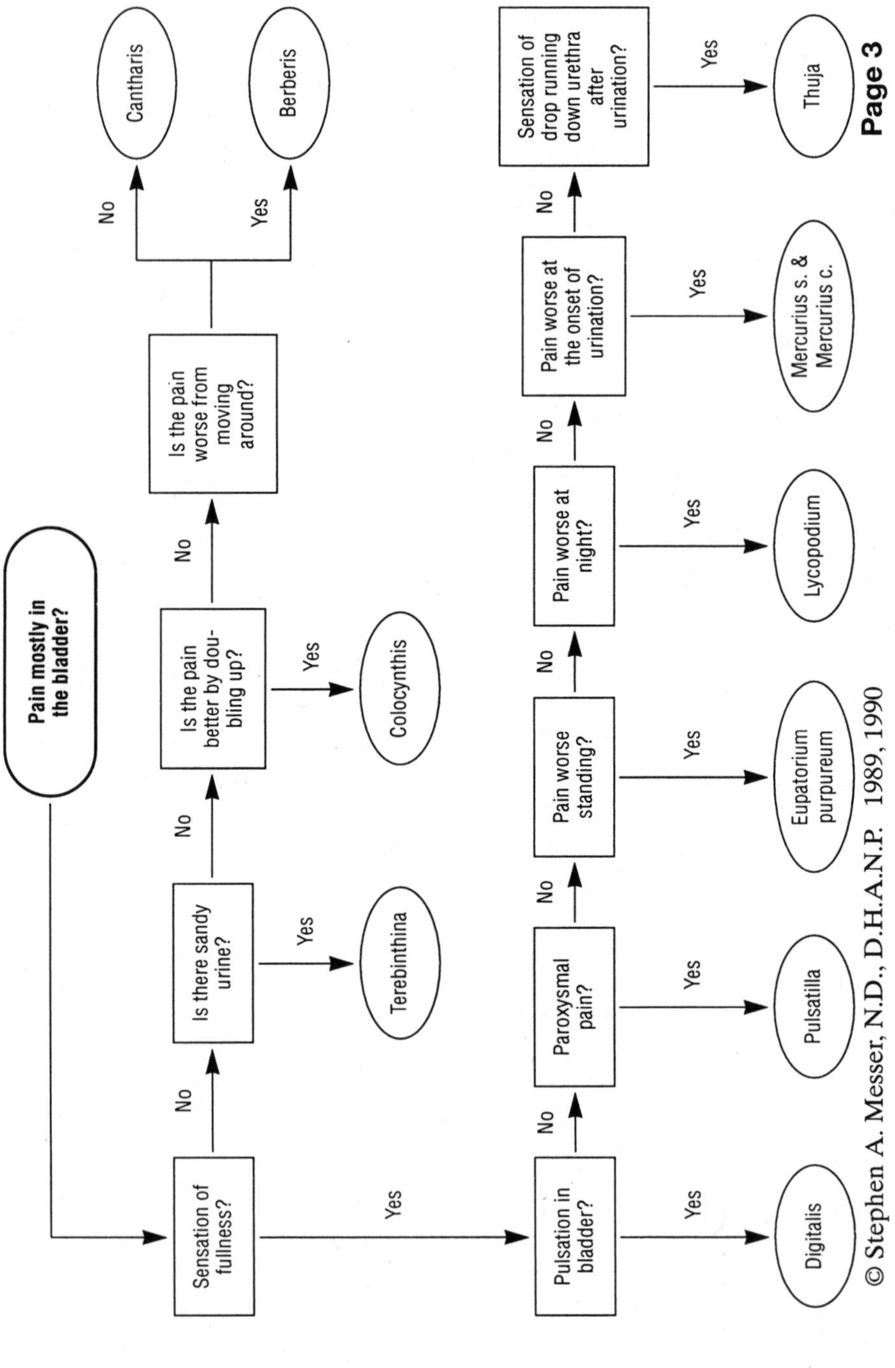

ACUTE OTITIS MEDIA

You diagnose acute otitis media in a child

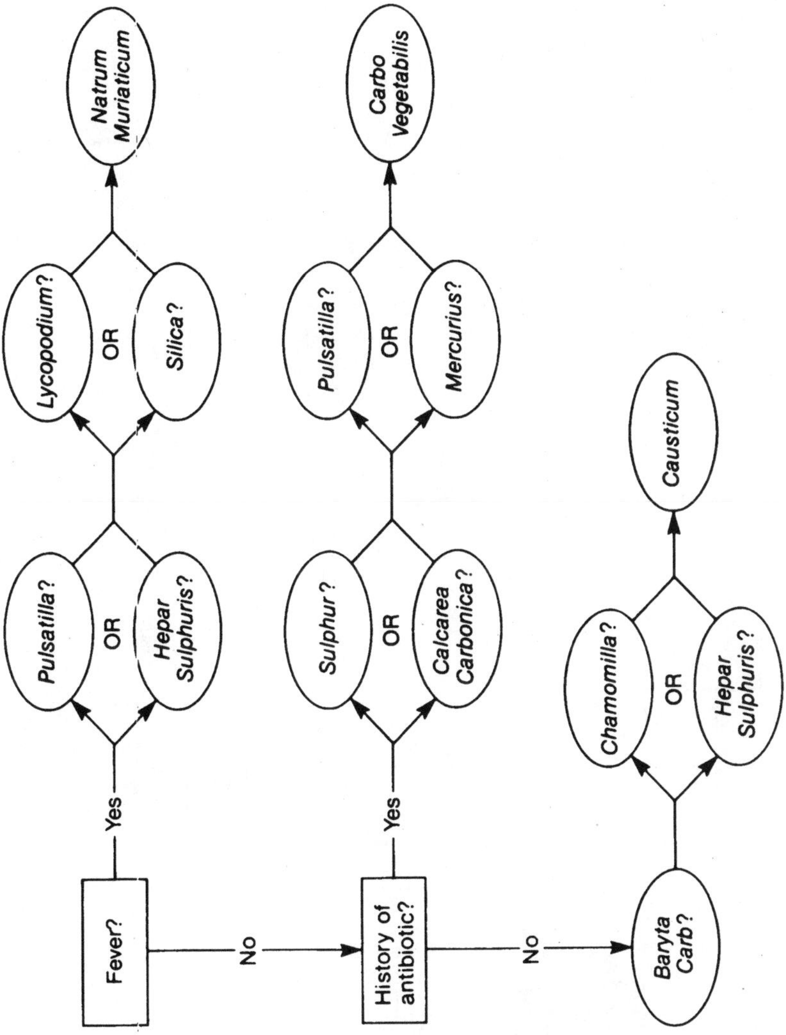

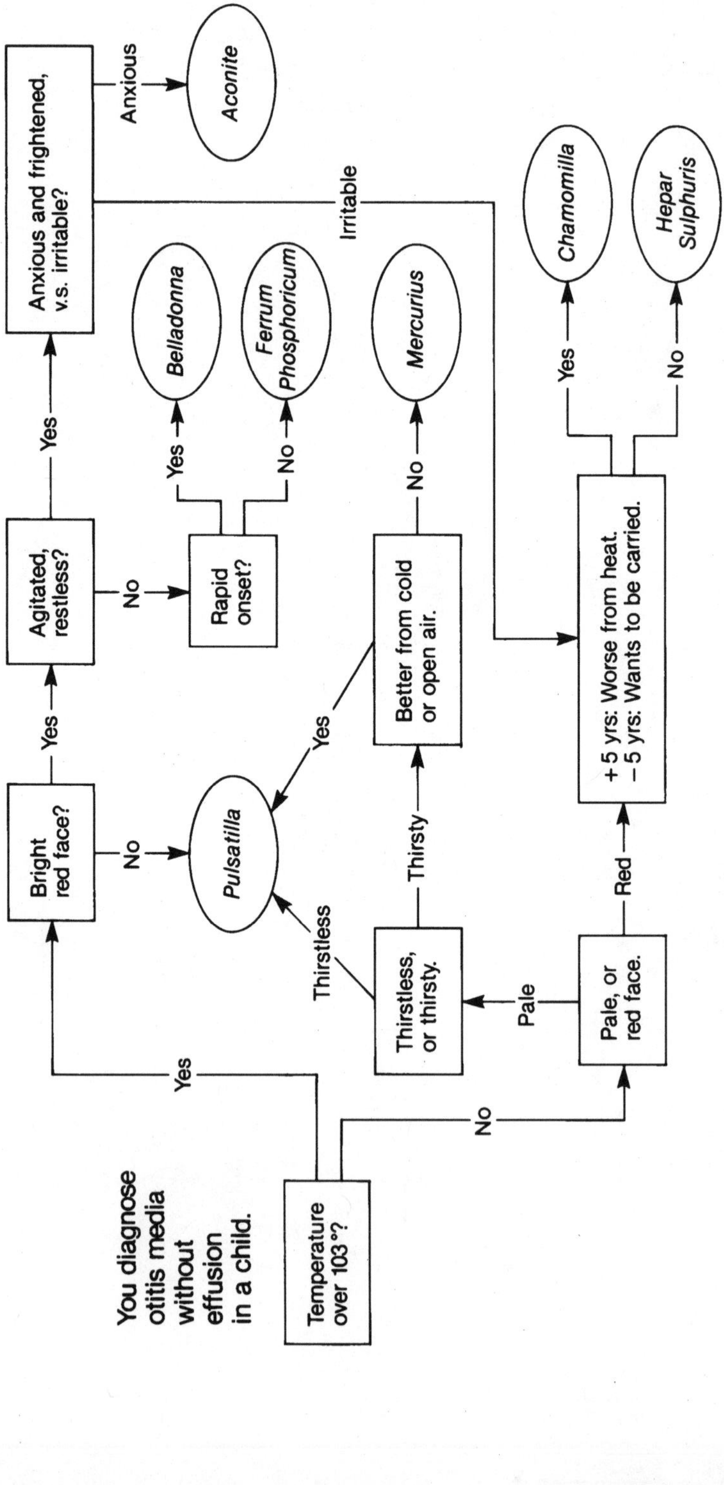
You diagnose otitis media without effusion in a child.
Temperature over 103°?
Yes
No
Bright red face?
Yes
No
Agitated, restless?
Yes
No
Anxious and frightened, v.s. irritable?
Anxious
Aconite
Irritable
Rapid onset?
Yes
No
Belladonna
Ferrum Phosphoricum
Pulsatilla
Pale, or red face.
Pale
Red
Thirstless, or thirsty.
Thirstless
Thirsty
Better from cold or open air.
Yes
No
Mercurius
+ 5 yrs: Worse from heat.
− 5 yrs: Wants to be carried.
Yes
No
Chamomilla
Hepar Sulphuris

INDEX—THERAPEUTIC

Dulcamara
Gnaphalium
Guaco
Guaiacum
Kali bic
Kali carb
Lachesis
Lycopodium
Natrum mur
Natrum sulph
Nux vomica
Oxalic acid
Phosphorus
Plumbum met
Rhus tox
Ruta
Silicea
Staphysagria
Sulphur
Tellurium
Thuja
Viscum album

BRONCHITIS

Aconite
Ammonium carb
Antimonium tart
Arsenicum alb
Balsam of Peru
Belladonna
Bryonia
Carbo veg
Conium
Drosera
Dulcamara
Ferrum phos
Hepar sulph
Ipecac
Mercurius
Natrum sulph
Phosphorus
Pulsatilla
Rumex
Sanguinaria
Senega
Spongia
Stannum

Also see Asthma/Pneumonia—Bronchial Lobar

BURNS

Arsenicum alb

Cantharis
Carbolic acid
Carbo veg
Causticum
Kreosotum
Urtica urens

Also see Wounds

CANKER SORES/ GLOSSITIS/ TRENCHMOUTH

Aethusa

Arsenicum alb
Baptisia
Borax
Cantharis
Kali chl
Lachesis
Mercurius cor
Mercurius sol
Mercurius viv
Muriatic acid
Natrum mur
Nitric acid
Nux vomica
Sulphur
Sulphuric acid

Tongue Inflammation

Antimonium crud

Apis
Crotalis c
Crotalis h

Gum Inflammation

Kreosotum
Petroleum
Phosphorus

CARDIAC PAIN/CHEST PAIN

Aconite
Cactus grand
Cenchris
Cereus b
Coffea
Digitalis
Gelsemium
Glonoine

Stramonium
Sulphur
Also see Laryngitis

CYSTITIS/INFLAMMATION OF THE BLADDER

Aconite
Apis
Arsenicum alb
Benzoic acid
Berberis
Cannabis indica
Cannabis sativa
Cantharis
Capsicum
Causticum
Equisetum
Lycopodium
Mercurius cor
Nux vomica
Pulsatilla
Sabina
Sarsaparilla
Sepia
Staphysagria
Terebinthina
Uva ursi
Also see Urethritis, Prostatitis

DIARRHEA/CHILDREN

Aconite
Aethusa
Arsenicum alb
Calcarea carb
Chamomilla
Colocynthis
Ipecac
Magnesia carb
Magnesia mur
Mercurius
Natrum sulph
Nux vomica
Podophyllum
Psorinum
Rheum
Stramonium
Sulphur
Also see Abdominal Inflammation, Colitis

DYSMENORRHEA

Belladonna
Borax
Bryonia
Cactus grand
Calcarea phos
Caulophyllum
Chamomilla
Cimicifuga
Colocynthis
Dioscorea
Graphites
Kali carb
Magnesia phos
Pulsatilla
Ustilago

EYE INJURIES/INFLAMMATION

Aconite
Arnica
Bothrops
Euphrasia
Hamamelis
Kalmia latifolia
Ledum
Mercurius cor
Naphthaline
Natrum mur
Osmium
Phosphorus
Pilocarpus
Pulsatilla
Rhus tox
Ruta
Staphysagria
Sulphur
Symphytum
Also see Conjunctivitis, Styes/Blepharitis, Wounds/Foreign Bodies

FLATULENCE

Argentum nit
Carbo veg
China
Colchicum
Lycopodium
Magnesia phos
Plumbum met

Phosphoric acid
Zincum met

Sick Headaches

Chelidonium
Cocculus
Iris
Nux vomica
Picric acid
Sulphur

Hormonal Headaches

Cyclamen
Graphites
Kreosotum
Pulsatilla
Sepia

HEAT STROKE/EXHAUSTION

Aconite
Amyl nitrite
Antimonium crud
Belladonna
Bryonia
Carbo veg
Gelsemium
Glonoine
Kali carb
Lachesis
Lycopodium
Natrum mur
Opium
Silicea

Also see Shock/Collapse

HEMORRHAGES

Arnica
Belladonna
Bothrops
Cantharis
Carbo veg
China
Crotalus h
Ferrum phos
Hamamelis
Ipecac
Lachesis
Melilotus
Mercurius
Millefolium
Nitric acid
Phosphorus
Sabina
Secale
Sulphuric acid

Also see Post Partum Bleeding, Wounds

HEMORRHOIDS

Aesculus
Aloe
Ammonium carb
Arsenicum alb
Carbo veg
Causticum
Collinsonia
Graphites
Hamamelis
Kali carb
Lachesis
Muriatic acid
Nitric acid
Nux vomica
Paeonia
Phosphorus
Pulsatilla
Ratanhia
Sepia
Sulphur
Teucrium

INFLUENZA

Aconite
Allium cepa
Arsenicum alb
Baptisia
Bryonia
Causticum
Eupatorium perf
Gelsemium
Hepar sulph
Influenzinum
Nux vomica
Oscillococcinum
Phosphoric acid
Pyrogen
Rhus tox
Scutellaria

Laurocerasus
Also see Shock/Collapse

Uterine Displacements

Aesculus
Aletris
Belladonna
Calcarea carb
Calcarea phos
Caulophyllum
Cimicifuga
Conium
Helonias
Kali carb
Lilium tig
Lycopodium
Mercurius
Murex
Natrum mur
Nux vomica
Phosphorus
Platina
Podophyllum
Pulsatilla
Ruta
Sepia

Retained Placenta

Belladonna
Cantharis
Cimicifuga
Gelsemium
Pulsatilla
Sabina
Secale
Sepia

Post Partum Hemorrhage

Aconite
Apocynum
Argentum nit
Arnica
Arsenicum alb
Belladonna
Bryonia
Calcarea carb
Cantharis
Carbo veg
Caulophyllum
Chamomilla
China
Cimicifuga
Crocus
Erigeron
Ferrum met
Ficus
Hamamelis
Hyoscyamus
Iodum
Ipecac
Kali carb
Lachesis
Lycopodium
Millefolium
Nitric acid
Nux moschata
Phosphorus
Platina
Pulsatilla
Sabina
Secale
Stramonium
Sulphur
Trillium
Ustilago
Also see Hemorrhages

Mastitis

Belladonna
Bryonia
Hepar sulph
Phosphorus
Phytolacca
Silicea
Also see Abscesses/Boils/Carbuncles

Lactation

Acetic acid
Borax
Lac caninum
Pulsatilla

Failure to Nurse

Aethusa

OTITIS MEDIA/EARACHES

Aconite
Bacillinum
Baryta carb
Belladonna
Calcarea carb

Capsicum
Carbo veg
Causticum
Chamomilla
Ferrum phos
Gelsemium
Hepar sulph
Hydrastis
Kali bic
Kali mur
Kali sulph
Lycopodium
Mercurius dulcis
Mercurius
Pulsatilla
Silicea
Sulphur
Tellurium

PELVIC INFLAMMATION//LEUKORRHEA

Aconite
Apis
Arsenicum alb
Belladonna
Cantharis
Cenchris
Colocynthis
Kreosotum
Lachesis
Lilium tig
Lycopodium
Medorrhinum
Mercurius
Nitric acid
Origanum
Platina
Pulsatilla
Rhus tox
Sabina
Sepia
Also see Abdominal Inflammation

PNEUMONIA/BRONCHIAL LOBAR

Aconite
Antimonium tart
Arsenicum alb
Bryonia
Calcarea carb
Carbo veg
Chelidonium
Ferrum phos
Ipecac
Kali carb
Lobelia
Lycopodium
Mercurius
Phosphorus
Pulsatilla
Rhus tox
Senega
Sepia
Silicea
Sulphur
Veratrum viride
Also see Asthma, Bronchitis

POISONING/FOOD

Agaricus
Arsenicum alb
Botulinum
Carbo veg
Cuprum ars
Pyrogen
Urtica urens
Also see Abdominal Inflammation, Diarrhea/Children, Nausea & Vomiting of Pregnancy

PROSTATITIS/PROSTATIC ENLARGEMENT

Apis
Baryta carb
Benzoic acid
Berberis
Calcarea carb
Cannabis indica
Chimaphilia
Clematis
Conium
Digitalis
Iodum
Lycopodium
Medorrhinum
Nitric acid
Pareira brava
Pulsatilla

Sabal serrulata
Selenium
Silicea
Spongia
Staphysagria
Sulphur
Thuja
Also see Cystitis/Bladder Inflammation, Urethritis

SHOCK/COLLAPSE

Aconite
Arnica
Camphor
Carbo veg
Cuprum met
Gelsemium
Nux moschata
Opium
Veratrum alb
Also see Heat Stroke/Exhaustion, Post Partum—APGAR

SINUSITIS

Arsenicum alb
Calcarea carb
Hydrastis
Kali bic
Mercurius
Natrum ars
Natrum carb
Natrum mur
Nux vomica
Oscillococcinum
Pulsatilla
Sepia
Silicea
Sulphur
Also see Headache/Congestive

SORE THROAT/PHARYNGITIS

Aconite
Ailanthus
Apis
Baryta mur
Belladonna
Cantharis
Dulcamara
Guaiacum
Hepar sulph
Kali bic
Lac caninum
Lachesis
Lycopodium
Mercurius cor
Mercurius cyan
Mercurius Iod Flav
Mercurius Iod Rub
Mercurius
Nitric acid
Phytolacca
Streptococcinum
Also see Laryngitis

STYES/BLEPHARITIS

Conium
Graphites
Lycopodium
Pulsatilla
Sepia
Silicea
Staphysagria
Sulphur
Also see Conjunctivitis, Eye Inflammation

URETHRITIS

Agnus castus
Alumina
Aurum met
Benzoic acid
Cannabis sativa
Cantharis
Cochlearia
Cubeba
Digitalis
Ferrum phos
Kali chl
Medorrhinum
Mercurius cor
Mercurius
Natrum sulph
Nitric acid
Petroselinum
Phosphoric acid
Pulsatilla
Selenium
Senecio

REMEDY INDEX